Politics and
Poetics of Migration

Politics and Poetics of Migration

NARRATIVES OF IRANIAN WOMEN
FROM THE DIASPORA

PARIN DOSSA

Canadian Scholars' Press Inc./Toronto

Politics and Poetics of Migration: Narratives of Iranian Women from the Diaspora
Parin Dossa

First published in 2004 by
Canadian Scholars' Press Inc.
180 Bloor Street West, Suite 801
Toronto, Ontario
M5S 2V6

www.cspi.org

Chapter 2, "Authored and Unauthored Texts," was originally published as "Narrative Mediation of Conventional and New 'Mental Health' Paradigms: Reading the Stories of Immigrant Iranian Women" in *Medical Anthropology Quarterly*, Vol. 16, No. 3: 341–359. © 2002 *American Anthropological Association*. Reprinted by permission of the University of California Press.

Chapter 3, "Being a Refugee in Canada: Sultan's Story," was originally published as "Reconfiguring the Question 'Who is a Refugee?' Coming to Voice, Coming to Power: One Woman's Story" in the *Pakistan Journal on Women's Studies: Alam-e-Niswan* Vol. 9, No. 1: 27–55. © 2002. Reprinted by permission of the publisher.

Chapter 4, "Looking for Work: Nadia's Story," was originally published as "Localized Impact of Global Restructuring of Work: Border-Crossing Stories of Iranian Women" in *Gender, Technology and Development* Vol. 7, No. 2: 209–232. © 2003 Sage Publications India Pvt. Ltd.

Every reasonable effort has been made to identify copyright holders. CSPI would be pleased to have any errors or omissions brought to its attention.

Canadian Scholars' Press gratefully acknowledges financial support for our publishing activities from the Government of Canada through the Book Publishing Industry Development Program (BPIDP) and the Government of Ontario through the Ontario Book Publishing Tax Credit Program.

National Library of Canada Cataloguing in Publication Data

Dossa, Parin Aziz, 1945-
    Politics and Poetics of Migration : narratives of Iranian women from the diaspora / Parin Dossa.

Includes bibliographical references and index.
ISBN 1-55130-272-1

    1. Iranian Canadian women—Mental health.   2. Women immigrants—Mental health—Canada.
3. Marginality, Social—Canada. 4. Displacement (Psychology)   5. Emigration and immigration—Psychological aspects.   I. Title.

FC106.I5D68 2004   305.48'96912'0971   C2004-900629-0

Typesetting: Brad Horning
Cover design: Up Inc
Author photo: Ron Long

06   07   08   5   4   3   2

Printed and bound in Canada by AGMV Marquis Imprimeur, Inc.

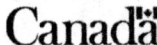

For Aziz

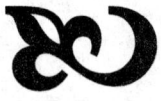

Table of Contents

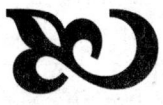

Acknowledgements

Politics and Poetics of Migration: Narratives of Iranian Women from the Diaspora has been for some time in the making, and it would not have been possible without the community of social justice activists, scholars and research participants in this study. For their generosity and commitment, I thank all the people whose words and actions gave form to this study. The good faith with which the participants created a space for me has left a deep imprint on my mind. Support and conversations with my Iranian colleagues Mahin Khodabandeh, Dr. Parvin Yavari and Roshi Ghomshei played a significant role in the development of this book. Mohammad Soufi and Forouzan Hassani were always ready with help and advice. During my brief stay in Iran, Ali Soofi and Nazi Sadeghzadeh offered their kind cooperation, for which I am grateful. My debts to all the contributors can never be repaid nor will they be forgotten. Special thanks go to Shabnam Ziabaksh and Poran Poregbal, who were my research assistants and who greatly enriched my understanding of the everyday lives of Iranian women. My thanks to Paridokht Anousheh for helping me to learn Farsi. I am also indebted to North Shore Multicultural Society, the Seniors Hub Centre, and North Shore Family Services for facilitating the progress of my research. The Canadian Council of Muslim Women made it possible for me to converse with Islamic scholars across Canada.

For support, critical insights and helpful suggestions I would like to thank many friends and colleagues, among them Gelya Frank, Isabel Dyck, Yasmin Jiwani, Sunera Thobani, Joan Anderson, Jo-Anne Lee, June Beynon and Habiba Zaman. Preliminary ideas for this study were commented on with care and thoughtfulness by Gelya

Frank. Special thanks to Joan Anderson for her perceptive response to parts of the book and to other anonymous reviewers for their invaluable comments. To Jo-Anne Lee, I would like to express my appreciation for the opportunity to dialogue. I am thankful to the many students I taught and learned from over many years.

My family has nurtured and sustained me in multiple ways. I thank Aziz for his love and companionship. He has expressed unfailing confidence in my work while constantly reminding me of the world beyond it. I thank my children, Fahreen and Zahwil, for bringing enormous joy and for the precious gift of parenting. For their affection and presence in my life, I thank my parents, Nabat and Umedali. My mother's love has been a source of strength and comfort.

A three-year research grant from the Social Science and Humanities Research Council of Canada to RIIM (The Vancouver Centre of Excellence in Research on Immigration and Integration in the Metropolis) enabled me to conduct this research. My special thanks go to the co-directors, Don De Voretz and David Ley, for their continual support and encouragement. The staff of Canadian Scholars' Press has been exemplary. I am indebted to Dr. Althea Prince, the managing editor, for her unwavering confidence in my work. Allyson Latta asked instructive questions and copyedited the manuscript meticulously, in the way that only she can. Thank you to Rebecca Conolly and Renée Knapp for their efficiency and hard work. With all the fine support I have received from the many individuals and organizations, any interpretative shortcomings are mine.

ONE

Introduction:
Epistemology and Methodology

There are several factors that affect our health such as good nutrition, good climate and not to have worries. I don't think I am a healthy person. I am lonely here and I don't have someone to talk to. It was better if I had someone to trust and talk about my concerns. (Sultan)

Someone who has peace in life, then the person is mentally healthy. (Nadia)

Every time I usually get depressed and I start to think about all different problems that we have and why we came here. As the time passed, our situation got worse. I feel like a prisoner. (Simin)

We came to Canada for a better quality of life. (Fatima)

We came to this county to work and unfortunately there are not any jobs and then we have to apply for welfare. The money they give us is not enough and they want us to get a roommate. I feel like a prisoner here. I am living with someone who makes me very angry all the time and I have to be home mostly as I don't have enough money to pay for transportation or go somewhere else for a few hours. (Razia)

I am going to Y college to study English. I am sitting in the same English class as the young girls and boys are sitting and teacher loaded us with lots of material which is too much for a woman

1

of my age [60 plus]. Last time I told myself that I am not going back to school. Teacher treats me the same with a 20-year-old person. But I decided to go back to school again. I cannot do anything without good English. If they accept immigrants, they have to produce work for them. Even I could not find two children to babysit. (Simin)

These are the words of women whose stories appear in the pages of this book. Part of a cohort of 47,000 post-revolution Iranian immigrants to British Columbia, the women settled on the North Shore in the 1980s and 1990s.[1] The newcomers came to experience what it is like to build a new life in a country where their citizenship rights remain undefined. Although Canada desires immigrants and refugees for their skills and for the way they enhance the country's international image as a humanitarian society, Iranian immigrants, like other racialized minorities, do not enjoy the Charter status accorded to the British and the French. As such they fall into the category of Other. For new immigrants, Othering translates into lack of opportunities and discrimination on a scale that violates their human rights and their sense of well-being (Agnew 1996, Bannerji 1995, Creese 1992, Dua 1999, Dyck 1995, Henry et al. 1995). Their "outsider" status, however, does not preclude the possibility of their showing "resistance" in ways that reveal both the fault lines of the dominant society and alternative ways of being—that is, creative adaptation to a new way of life in Canada. *Politics and Poetics of Migration: Narratives of Iranian Women from the Diaspora* is the story of post-revolution Iranian migrants as seen primarily through the eyes of four women. Each life represents a particular social location that brings into relief the complex ways in which individuals experience and rework migration and resettlement in the context of everyday life.

The experiences of post-revolution Iranian immigrants may be understood within the rubric of social suffering. Drawing upon insights from Das and Kleinman (2001) and Kleinman et al. (1997), I argue that social suffering is a multi-faceted phenomenon. At one level, it involves the impact of social, economic and global capitalism on the everyday lives of people. Yet this is not the end point.

Insensitive bureaucratic and institutional responses intensify the impact of social suffering in ways that normalizes it. Furthermore, by deploying powerful discourses and practices, institutions make themselves immune from criticism and scrutiny. But there is another side of the story, revealing that suffering cannot be subject to total appropriation, management and control. The process of marginalization generates alternative discourses, and sufferers continue to give voice to their concerns using multiple means of expression, including even the silent language of the body. Life stories, such as those of the women in this book, also constitute a powerful medium of communication. Although discursive in nature, stories lend texture to macro-level analysis.

In short, an examination of social suffering, as Chuengsatiansup has noted, helps us to understand both the painful experiences of "those whose social existence has been excluded, discounted, dehumanized, and displaced by the dominant political discourse" (2001, 32) and the ways in which those on the periphery can challenge the dominant centre.

How do we acquire a concrete and palpable understanding of the impact of the social forces on individuals and communities? How do we address the paradox of perpetuation of affliction by institutions established to relieve suffering in the first place? How do we speak with and not for our research participants so as to recognize them as "producers of knowledge"? What role does storytelling play in creating "a world that we ought to know," to use Razack's (1998) words? How do researchers "witness" suffering as opposed to merely observing it? These questions guided my analysis of the narratives that I was privileged to hear during the course of my research on the North Shore, from September 1997 to April 2001.

"Were it not for the Iranian revolution, we would not be in Canada" was one comment that was commonly expressed. While each of the women to whom I talked presented her unique version of the revolution, the script of foreign intervention was collectively spelled out. As one woman expressed it, [Britain and the United States came to Iran to get our oil. But they never left." In Iran, though the country was not formally colonized, the influence of the West in shaping its political life was strong and had to be reckoned with at multiple levels: social, economic and discursive.] More poignantly,

3

as the participants were aware, the process of displacement and dislocation does not come to an end upon immigration but may continue in the country of settlement, resulting in unnecessary suffering. This is brought to light through the words of the women cited at the beginning of this chapter.

Displacement is an embodied experience that invariably reflects the workings of the dominant system. Yet, paradoxically, in a world where categories and classification matter, this dominant system has the authority to label displaced people as anomalous. Without this hegemonic topography that defines nation-states, we cannot institute what Malkki refers to as "a powerful regime of order and knowledge" (1995, 8). Displaced people are seen as challenging and subverting this order and this is why national and international bodies control and manage anyone who is perceived not to have territorial roots. A common strategy is to use the idiom of mental health, as exemplified in constructs such as "refugee mental health" and "post-traumatic stress disorder." As experienced by study participants, these powerful constructs led social service providers to frame what were in fact social and economic concerns in medical terms: "They are stressed"; "They cannot adjust to our way of life"; "They bring their cultural baggage with them"; "They are depressed." Such a discourse barely implicates the system and thus the cause-and-effect relationship between health, and our societal institutions, practices, norms and values appears severed.

The social experiences of the women in my study included their surviving the Iranian Revolution, dealing with Canadian immigration and refugee policies that determine "who gets in," migrating and re-settling, coping with everyday reality, and reconstructing new lives in the wake of multiple social barriers. I show that these women's attempts to make sense of their suffering include relating their displacement and resettlement narratives.

With this context in mind I have placed several individual Iranian immigrant women and their stories at the centre of my study. My goal is to bring to the fore a politically grounded understanding of social suffering as exemplified on the plane of displacement and societal issues.

Note that immigrant women's voices on mental health (read: societal issues) have often been silenced. Policy makers, service providers and medical practitioners alike render these women socially invisible. The challenge is to listen to the voices in a manner that allows us to capture the lived reality of the speakers while simultaneously understanding how systems of domination and unequal power relations shaped this reality. Ultimately the task at hand is to recognize these women as producers of knowledge. Only at this level can we understand the extent to which socioeconomic forces are implicated in their suffering. At a deeper level, we must *converse* with the women (dialogical mode) and not *speak* with them (appropriation mode). The following sections explain how I came to map the lives of immigrant Iranian women during the course of my research.

Treading a Fine Line
ೞ

As I undertook this study, I immediately found three challenges. First, in keeping with the tenor of ethnographic research, I wanted to identify a field site that would allow me to work with participants over an extended period. Such a focus, as I show below, made it possible for me to look at displacement as a process rather than a given fact—a point that needs emphasis in the wake of the powerful Eurocentric script where displacement is an event that occurs elsewhere, "out there" in other spaces. Second, I wanted to look at the concept of mental health to further explore the paradox spelled out by medical anthropologists: mental health is an embodied experience, yet it is the professional categories that determine who is "sick" (Kleinman et al. 1997, Dyck 1998). Third, I wanted to create a forum for a multi-voiced dialogue that would act as a point of intervention into the hegemonic constructs of "refugee mental health" or "mental health of displaced people" (Ong 1995b). It is necessary to reverse the current process in which the sufferer, in a situation of powerlessness, is compelled to take on the burden of affliction. The sufferer's body is referred to as diseased and in need of cure, albeit in isolation. The sociopolitical script is thereby suppressed, but not totally. As Das et al. (2000) have informed us, the sufferers reconstruct and remake their worlds despite tremendous odds. These newly created forms, as Bonny (2000) notes, cannot be specified in mechanical or structural terms but in terms of relationships and culture-in-the-making.

The way I framed my research project and addressed the above issues may be described as ethnographic narrative.[3] I define *ethnographic narrative* as a mode of research embedded in multi-voiced dialogue where research participants have central space. As such, the participants speak to multiple audiences: service and health professionals, researchers, readers and peers. In this regard, it is useful to consider ethnographic narrative as a text-in-the-making and as "active." Dorothy Smith refers to this process as being one in which participants are like speakers in a conversation—"present and active," in her terms, in speaking to us. Produced by one or more people in actual settings, the text constitutes a "part of a course of action, whether of an individual, a group, an organization of some kind or an extended social relation concerning the activities of many. And its reading also is in time and actual place and enters again into someone's course of action and has, in that course of action, a speaking part; it becomes active in that course of action" (1999, 135–136). In a similar vein, Gelya Frank has noted: "When readers engage with the life story [the text] and its various interpretations, new meanings are created that will reverberate in the readers' own local cultures and sometimes the dominant culture as well (2000, 23). Multi-voiced dialogue may nest between conventional categories that shape our taken-for-granted reality. This is especially the case with refugees. Krulfeld and Camino state:

> In such positions of liminality and marginality, all aspects of their [refugees] lives are called into question, including ethnic and national identity, gender roles, social relationships and socio-economic status. Such liminality does not, however, abruptly begin at the point at which refugees leave their homes, but is rather founded in the turmoil of their lives even before flight and resettlement continuing during the search for asylum and relocation. (1994, x)

My first task was to identify participants willing to share their experiences of displacement and resettlement. As I considered attaining mental health to be an integral part of this process, I did not seek out participants with particular health issues. I contacted a number of service organizations, which then put me in touch with several Iranian women. Among my criteria was that the women had to have migrated to Canada over the last ten years to fifteen years. This time span allowed me to look at mental health and resettlement as processes rather than reified occurrences. With the help of two Iranian research assistants, I interviewed fifteen women from the North Shore, home of the majority of the Iranians in metropolis Vancouver. I too lived on the North Shore at the time of this study. Four of the women shared their life narratives in full over a period of two to two-and-a-half years. Each participant was interviewed for one-and-a-half to two hours, over one to three sittings. The interviews were taped, translated and transcribed. In addition, I talked to several dozen women during the course of my ethnographic research at different sites, especially at the Mall Walking Program— a recreation programme whereby senior citizens meet regularly and exercise by walking in a shopping mall—and an English-as-a-second-language (ESL) class. Insights from this data informed my analysis of the narratives presented in this study.

From 1997 to 1998, my assistants and I participated in the Mall Walking Program along with Iranian seniors (as clients) and younger Iranian women and men (as service providers). We invited the participants of this programme to be part of the research project and developed a semi-structured questionnaire for discussion. From December 1999 to March 2000, I also helped to run an ESL/Mental Health support programme that gave me background on a wide range of issues—life in Iran, family life, jobs, training programmes, racism, women's concerns, and Iranian festivals—all of which Iranian adult learners discussed in an open and participatory learning environment.

I had originally planned to include data from all the interviews. However, as the study progressed I began to see patterns in women's responses: there were some women who shared full stories of their lives; others were content to give what they regarded as basic information, often prefacing their vignettes with the words "One Iranian woman's story is everyone's story." This form of testimonial response led me to focus on the stories of four women, all of whom shared their stories with me with the hope that they could be written up in full as narrative texts that they had "authored." Except for one woman of Baha'i faith, all interviewees were Shi'a Muslim—the majority religion in Iran and a minority sect within Islam. Two of the women (Nadia and Fatima) read and commented on the transcripts; the other two (Sultan and Zahra) were happy to have the opportunity to tell their stories. Nadia and Fatima are bilingual and their preferred choice of language was English. (My presence may have prompted them to use English because I do not speak Farsi.[4]) The other two narrators spoke Farsi, and their interview texts were later transcribed and translated by a research assistant. Women were encouraged to use the language of their choice, and six out of the other eleven women spoke in English while the rest used Farsi. Formal interviews and storytelling sessions were conducted at various sites: mall and strip mall cafeterias, my home and ESL classes. I have fictionalized all names, and changed any information, for example professional background or workplace, that would reveal participants' identities.

The order in which I arranged the stories is determined by two criteria: the *what*, or focus, of the story and the *how*, or way, it is related. In this regard, the first two stories provide a collective context (what) for the lives of post-revolution Iranian women: being a refugee/displaced (Sultan) and looking for work (Nadia). The last two stories focus on the use of particular tools (how), such as silence and metaphors, that the women use to voice their concerns. Zahra's and Fatima's stories on aging/life course and caregiving, respectively, show that speaking in itself is a reflexive and politicized act, and both women were keen to ensure that their stories were heard in order to effect change. The ground-clearing chapter (Chapter 2) captures the collective voices of these women and explains both the what and the how of their storytelling.

Ethnography
ಬಌ

Only in the last few decades have anthropologists paid close attention to ethnographic writing. Prior to the problematization of the ethnographic text, the data were considered as a set and were converted from their original form (seen as strange and irregular facts) into familiar and orderly text for consumption by a professional community. After being in the field for over three years and actively collecting data, especially during my annual research semesters, I had accumulated a substantive set. I had life narrative and interview/ vignettes data, data from my diary entries, newspaper clippings, as well as data from participant observations. My next step was to organize these data in a way that would help me to understand the intricate ways in which women reworked the dominant discourses on displacement and mental health.

The challenge, then, is not the documentation of empirical evidence but epistemological concerns: what is social knowledge for, how is it produced, and for whom? A multi-faceted approach to the presentation of data constitutes one response. Taking a cue from Norton (2000), I present the data as descriptive, analytical (my particular reading of the text) and interpretive (drawing upon the literature), interactively, without drawing boundaries. To some extent the data speak for themselves through the narrative scripts of women; in some cases, I have analyzed the data to foster dialogue. In other cases, I acknowledge my role in interpreting the data by drawing upon relevant literature.

How I Came to Study Mental Health
ೞ

When I began my fieldwork in the fall of 1997, "mental health" among Iranian immigrant women was an area that called for attention. Service providers and policy makers had adopted the popular script that attributed Iranian women's (homogeneously constructed) mental health problems to experiences of displacement that occurred because of the chaos prevailing in their own country. Iranian women perceived the situation differently. They were engaged in articulating a politicized script that implicated societal factors for their emotional distress. Through my research I learned that these women did not resort to presenting a laundry list of issues: lack of English training classes, downward professional mobility, and institutional and systemic racism. To express their concerns, women chose to tell the stories of their lives on the grounds, as mentioned earlier, that "one woman's story is everyone's story." This dynamic is captured by Patricia Hill Collins who, in linking her personal odyssey with that of other African-American women, notes that "the voice that I now seek is both individual and collective, personal and political, one reflecting the intersection of my unique biography with the larger meaning of my historical times" (2000: xii).

My early fieldwork experiences brought home the point that we work towards a broader understanding of mental health—one that goes beyond the biomedical model to include women's own understandings (experiences and potential solutions) on this subject. This means establishing narrative points of intervention into the hegemonic script that erases crucial differences of gender, race and class and holds people responsible for their suffering. These women's own takes on displacement and alternative ways of framing the reality of their lives are not wholly derived from Western epistemology; neither are they confined within the unit of a discrete culture. As Moore expresses it:

> Indigenization of knowledge(s) while potentially powerfully creative for individuals and collectivities within specific contexts, runs the risk of defining certain kinds of knowledge as absolutely local, without comparative scope or wider application. It is imperative that anthropology should recognize that local knowledge, including local technical knowledge, can be part of a set of local knowledges properly pertaining to political economy and the social sciences, and can be comparative in scope as well as international in outlook. (1996, 6)

The issue of alternative epistemologies deserves more attention and hence I will consider what my home discipline of anthropology/medical anthropology has to say on the subject.

Medical anthropology has the potential to address the issue of what makes us human at a broader and more profound level because health, illness and displacement are concerns that we share cross-culturally, temporally and in space. This is because human suffering and distress transcend established "dichotomies of theory and practice, thought and action, objectivity and subjectivity" (Lindenbaum and Lock 1993, x). Towards this end, medical anthropology has demystified and revealed the culturally constructed nature of biomedicine, which has presented itself as "natural." This venture has been made possible through the analysis of data drawn from non-Western societies. But this orientation has created a gap between Western and non-Western medical systems. Ironically, examining the "irrational" systems of the non-Western world allows the much-needed critique of the seemingly "rational" system of Western biomedicine. Conventionally, medical anthropologists have attempted to explain the "irrationality" of other systems by demonstrating that they make sense in their own cultures, thus reinforcing the parent discipline's conventional orientation of Othering.

Like biomedicine, medical anthropology has entered into specialized fields, such as mental health (understood along a continuum of depression and mental illness), AIDS, chronic illness, disability and other conditions framed under the rubric of "illness." These ever-proliferating disease categories bring to the fore the gap between theory and practice. Does suffering lead to a more humane understanding of life or does it accentuate social markers of difference such as gender, age, race and disability? If illness brings us closer to understanding the humanness of our condition, how do we identify the parameters of the interconnections? This situation is complicated by the fact that the West has presented itself as the repository of "humane" values. If we claim that there are different ways of being human, how do we communicate and understand our differences and at the same time find common ground for interactive encounters? Search for these answers involves a long journey where we can only take a few steps at a time. I present my research as a few first steps in a journey that is long and arduous.

In the course of my field research, I realized that immigrant Iranian women have a lot to say on the subject of "mental health." And their understanding is politicized. The women that I talked to had a good understanding of the linkage between the social conditions of their lives and their well-being. "Why is it so difficult for us to find work?" "Why is it so difficult for us to access job- and language-training programmes?" "Why are we treated as 'different'?" Their narratives evoked further questions, such as the following: What was life like back at home? What is it like to be displaced?

How can one maintain a sense of well-being when powerful institutions—health/biomedicine, welfare, legal and others—erase and appropriate one's lived reality? These questions embedded in storied lives inform my analysis of the data.

Women's stories suggest that wellness is an integral part of the process of reconstructing lives and recapturing meaning in a new land. This focus allows me to address two interrelated issues. First, displacement, human suffering and health, as these come to light through narratives and historical trajectories as well as through institutional and social relationships, form part of the human condition across cultures. Health affects us all, and it is the search for human striving for well-being that has been the inspirational force for me. Travel along this path is challenging as our encounters are governed by socio-economic differences. The scenario is clear: Ours is a divided world where the distinction between the Western and the non-Western world is sharp. At issue is not only the material conditions of life but epistemological orientations through which the West constructs itself in relation to the Other. The Other is what the West is *not*. To complicate matters, the Other must be part of the Western landscape, a means through which the Other (read: inferior) can legitimize and reinforce the West's assumed superior status. The West has maintained its position discursively and otherwise by presenting itself as the upholder of values of "democracy" and "freedom" that in actual fact are available only to some people. Its gendered and racial script has been well laid out: democracy and freedom are first and foremost the prerogative of white males (Bannerji 2000, Lee and Cardinal 1998).

Second, in a world where asymmetrical relationships of power determine the availability of health and social resources, it is necessary to examine health and illness issues from the lived reality of racialized and displaced people. This point is especially important in light of the fact that the have-nots are increasingly constructed as a dependent population in need of aid and therapy. These seemingly humane forms of interventions, as Waters (2001) argues, lead to a structural rupture where the privileged are seen to be helping those Others rather than acknowledging their role in creating conditions that marginalize people in the first place. Institutional responses are oblivious to indigenous voices that have much to contribute to our understanding of the workings of political economy as well as the making of a just world. These voices will help us to resolve the efficiency-versus-quality-of-care dilemma in which our health and social systems have been embroiled. Our point of intervention then must be at a level where displaced women are recognized as producers of knowledge—a task that I undertake through the genre of storytelling.

Mapping the Path of Research
∾

For anyone doing research on immigrant communities, there are a number of issues that need careful reflection. The first one concerns the demarcation of the socio-cultural and racialized boundary of the community in question. How do we research communities and talk to individual members who are connected with what Appadurai (1991) refers to as ethnoscapes—the shifting and ever-changing landscapes of people connected to multiple social and cultural traditions? A critical issue here is to acknowledge that cultural and religious minorities engage with the larger society, a point that is overlooked in our concern to research discrete and socially constructed communities. When it comes to research on mental health, we are compelled to deal with epistemological formulations that cannot easily be addressed. Here we are in the realm of the hegemony of biomedicine that has determined the parameters of illness presented as universal and objective. Furthermore biomedicine with its tradition of reductionism (Lock 1993) does not address issues of well-being and health. Its focus is diagnoses of illness. Towards this end I deploy the narrative genre, which in essence provides insights into how life worlds are reinterpreted and reconfigured. This form of reconfiguration, as noted above, contains a dialogical component that, in the case of the Iranian women (post-revolution migrants), includes a collective story—the *testimonio*.

For people fleeing from a revolution, as was the case with my participants, there is a collective story that Beverley refers to as testimonio. Testimonio has two characteristics: it suggests both an urgency to communicate a problem and a need to articulate "a problematic collective social situation in which the narrator lives. The situation of the narrator in testimonio is one that must be representative of a social class or group" (1992, 95).

The sense of dislocation expressed through the idiom of mental health has been noted in the literature. Social service organizations are cognizant of this issue and have begun to address this concern by taking into account the vulnerability of the immigrant population, especially the elderly and women. However, there exists a wide gap between the social service discourse on mental health and the actual strategies deployed by populations to maintain their health and well-being. By and large, service organizations use the medical model: mental health is understood in terms of illness symptoms, the social/ proactive remedy for which is sought in recreational programmes (drop-in centres and some social activities) put into place with limited and fluctuating resources. The medical model has limited or no space to accommodate the viewpoints of "patients"; nor is it geared towards establishing connections with diverse communities (Anderson and Kirkham 1998).

Given these issues, my first task was to establish a relationship with the participants at a level where they are recognized as producers of knowledge in their own right, a topic that has received some attention in the works of critical and feminist anthropologists (Frank 2000, Wolf 1996, Smith 1999). In *Feminist Dilemmas in Fieldwork*, for example, Dianne Wolf articulates the issue in this way: "What kind of dilemmas, quandaries and contradictions have feminists confronted and grappled with in the process of fieldwork and its aftermath?" Wolf suggests that activism and consciousness-raising constitute one medium through which we can subvert the power hierarchy between the privileged researcher and her subjects; demystifying the notion of [Western] feminism as an all-encompassing home for all women and feminists is another medium (Anderson 1991). On a second note, Henrietta Moore raises this question: "What is social knowledge for?" She suggests that this question does not require a response but a series of interrogations "along the lines of what sort of knowledge is produced, for whom and for what reason" (1996, 2).

Our first point of entry must be that of location of our positions as researchers. Who we are and what motivates us to undertake research at particular sites are issues that must be contextualized so as to locate "the agency of the anthropologist within the same frame as the agency of the others, and thus to develop new forms of social engagement that ensure a radical departure from the earlier situations of anthropologists speaking for the others" (Moore 2000, 15). In this spirit I present my own story that speaks to the rupturing of cultural traditions and languages.

Search for Subaltern Knowledge
ಐ

I was born in what was colonial Uganda into a Shi'a Muslim family with ancestral links to India. My education was polarized. Officially, we were exposed to the colonial British system of education, which translated into marginalization of my "home" cultures and languages. It was my birthright to learn Gujerati (my mother tongue), Arabic and Farsi (Islamic), and Swahili (the language of my "host" country). This cultural wealth, however, remained largely inaccessible, being confined to the discreet sphere of home and community. During the early years of my education, we were subject to corporeal punishment (ruler on the knuckles) for speaking in any language but English. We were told that English was the language of civilization and to not speak it was detrimental to our "progress" in a rapidly changing world of "science and technology." In history and geography we learned about the accomplishments of the British Empire and the ways in which it had rescued its colonial subjects from dark ages. Exemplary literature, we were taught, was found primarily in the works of British writers.

A major paradox was that growing up in East Africa meant knowing next to nothing about African history, geography, literature, art and culture. Only peripheral space was given to these subjects and that even at a time when Uganda, Kenya and Tanzania were about to become independent nation-states (1960s). Islam and its rich international heritage was also subject to marginalization. In other words, other heritages were only brought into the picture to highlight the point that they were "undeveloped" and therefore would benefit from the civilizing mission of the West. The result of distorted curriculum is well summed up by Althea Prince: "... the teaching of distorted history, or history isolated into a series of interpreted pieces of information, can effectively distort a people's whole existence" (2001, 75).

Ugandan Asian Muslims, like other Asian minorities, were constrained by the colonial system. To begin with, the British confined the Asians (regarded as a homogenous category) to towns and small trading settlements, where they were channelled into trade: "Any non-African found living or trading outside a gazette township commits an offence" (Fernando 1979). The positioning of the Asians into the vulnerable middle status of being below the Europeans but economically above the Africans planted seeds of animosity. The frustration of the Africans arising from exploitation of their labour and their material resources (raw products) was levelled directly at the Asians. In 1972, President Idi Amin expelled all Ugandan Asians (Muslims, Hindus, Sikhs and other groups) from the country. Lives built over three generations came to end within the span of 90 days—the time period given to the Asians to leave.

At this moment in time I began to understand the political economy of displacement—the rupturing of relations wrought by colonization—a point brought home to me through the split forced upon our family. My parents and younger brother were sent to a refugee camp in England, while the Canadian immigration office made arrangements for my sister and me to come to Canada. I shared the kind of moment captured by the Chilean refugee writer:

> When she realized that she was surrounded by nothingness, she wanted to hug her own body, only now she realized that her body was the hole and the hole was her. The only clear thing in the midst of total darkness was her voice, trapped in her throat, trying to remember how to cry out for help ... but, in what language? (Rodriguez 1997, 35)

My Iranian informants often posed the following question to me: "How is it that you have found such a nice job in Canada and we are not able to do the same?" My immediate response was that I have been in Canada for a longer period and that I have in fact struggled like other immigrants. But on further reflection, I would suggest that I have paid a price to be where I am and this price is the loss of a rich heritage erased by the soft knife of politics. The pressure of having to fit into the dominant system at the expense of suppressing your own heritage is captured by Hill Collins:

> Oppressed groups ideas are frequently placed in the situation of being listened to only if we frame our ideas in the language that is familiar to and comfortable for a dominant group. This requirement often changes the meaning of our ideas and works to elevate the ideas of dominant groups. (1990, xiii)

It is this loss and suppression of rich heritages that has served as a catalyst for this work. Hence, a search for an alternative and interventionist epistemology—not to be understood as a discrete sphere—forms the mainstay of this work. I have chosen women's stories on displacement and mental health as a medium to articulate the contours of this epistemology at a particular moment in time. The issue here is this: How do we listen so that the women who speak are recognized as engaged participants (read: not victims) working through but also going beyond socially created suffering?

Taking the example of Black women, Hill Collins argues that new knowledge can emerge if we place women's everyday experiences and ideas at the centre of our analysis. Citing her own example, she notes: "Initially I found the movement between my training as an 'objective' social scientist and my daily experiences as an African-American woman jarring. But reconciling what we have been trained to see as opposites ... was freeing for me" (1990, xiv). She argues that within these new spaces that transcend the either-or scenario, women's voices are heard (also refer to Ong 1995a).

Storytelling
❧

In the last two decades, storytelling has been given centre stage in the works of anthropologists and feminist scholars globally. This genre's potential for bottom-up research has been noted and recognized. But as is the case with any kind of methodology, in its unexamined form it can be appropriated by dominant groups. Najmabadi's (1998b) work on the story of the daughters of Quchan, an Iranian village, provides an illustrative example. She shows that the daughters' stories of abduction were inscribed into the national imagination of the country not for the purpose of redress but to serve political ends of the constitutional revolution in progress (1900–1912). Taking the example of the refugee hearing process in Canada, Razack (1998) argues that unless displaced women present themselves as oppressed by the patriarchal cruelty of their families, communities or nations, they are not heard and asylum is not granted. The victimization stories of these women, according to Razack, serve to perpetuate the epistemological binary between the non-Western world and the West. The West, in positioning itself as superior, capitalizes on the construction of the non-West as barbaric and cruel to its women. Overlooked here is the colonial legacy of exploitation that creates asylum seekers—social sufferers—in the first place (Harrison 1997, Razack 1998).

The issue then is that unless women's stories serve to advance patriarchal and imperialist interests, they are not heard and their stories do not make their way into the national and the international corridors of power. In an attempt to create a space where women's stories are valorized as genuine attempts towards reinterpreting and remaking the worlds in which they live, narrative scholars have identified a number of critical and reflexive perspectives.

Anthropologist Gelya Frank suggests that gathering information on a life story must be accompanied by "a methodology in action as a source of primary data" (2000, 22). This stance, she argues, allows us to see how the biographical self is influenced by and also influences a particular cultural milieu over time. Frank observes that if stories are listened to in an appropriate way they have the potential to effect social change. This is due to the fact that when readers of these stories engage with them and their various interpretations, new meanings are created that will reverberate in the readers' own local culture and sometimes the dominant culture as well.

Anthropologist Julie Cruikshank (1998) notes that one route we can follow to ensure that stories of marginalized people are heard is to analyze how translation occurs across boundaries. This focus, she argues, breathes new life into stories as it creates greater appreciation of how the stories can be retrieved and reintroduced in new contexts. The aspect of new contexts is well summarized by Razack (1998), who notes that the stories of marginal groups reveal the world that we ought to know. In this vein, I want to suggest that listening is not a linear process; to grasp the meaning of the content and the manner in which stories are related requires second and third readings, which anchor stories in the larger social-political context. This form of contextualized reading makes it possible for us to challenge the us–them boundaries and question the validity of our taken-for-granted world. Razack has expressed it thus: Inasmuch as they capture the world of people who have experienced pain and suffering, the stories of marginalized people are bound to suggest knowledge of a just world (Ibid.; also see Dossa 2002).

Stories are also social as they reveal the complex ways in which individuals are interconnected with the world, a microcosm of which is the communities in struggle. Yet, in the West, liberal democracy is premised on the fact that "an individual is thought to be an autonomous, rational self, essentially unconnected to other selves and dedicated to pursuing his or her own interests" (Razack 1998, 38), thereby severing the individual from society.

Within the discipline of anthropology, narratives (storytelling) have achieved a level of theoretical and methodological sophistication. Gelya Frank, for example, identifies reflexivity as an important principle that addresses the charge that research on less privileged women can be potentially exploitative. The principle of reflexivity allowed Frank to ask questions that are barely considered in research: "How I came to understand Diane, how working with her transformed my understanding of her life, and how our collaboration may have influenced the life story Diane has to tell" (2000, 2).

Addressing the concerns of betrayal in field research, Aihwa Ong cautions us not to assume that subjects of our research are devoid of power and agency. For us to recognize this, Ong argues, we need to have a more complex understanding of power understood as "a decentralized, shifting and productive force, animated in networks of relations rather than possessed by individuals" (1995a, 353). This stance, according to Ong, is vitally significant as it enables our subjects to be part of the "cultural conversations in metropolitan centres"—a location that gives central space to people who are otherwise relegated to the margins. Re-examined notions of reflexivity and power are of value as it is within these spaces that we can foster progressive dialogue.

The above discussion establishes one point: stories and narratives have the potential to effect social change provided they form part of the larger political, social, historical, cultural and literary landscapes of societies. The possibility of the displaced Iranian women becoming part of the Canadian landscape is remote, as their structural and social exclusion is intense. Yet their stories must be heard if we want to write a different kind of Canadian history: a history where women from different cultural and linguistic backgrounds have an active presence. As Trinh has expressed it: "It will take a long time, but the story must be told" (1989, 119). Our listening must then be active, and directed to the process of coming to know about the lives of those who tell their stories and what we do with the stories once we have heard them. One thing that we must not do is appropriate stories of suffering.

Establishing a Paradigm of Telling and Listening
❧

> But listening or reading are not passive, neutral activities. We engage in a dialogue, whether we are in an actual conversation with another person, or watching the television, or reading a newspaper. While we read or listen, we continually make judgments about what we see or hear; we make sense through a process of selection and rejection. And what we select and reject very much depends on who we are, who is speaking to us, what they say, how they say it, where and when we are listening. (Casey 1993, 7)

My choice of storytelling with its potential for dialogue may appear to be anomalous in a world dominated by racist oppression, gender inequality and class disparities. Yet an analysis of only power and domination leads to victimization of the oppressed. Critical scholarship has enabled us to identify processes and structures that dominate and exploit. But this body of work has not substantially advanced paradigms of change that incorporate the viewpoints of oppressed groups. Stories provide one point of intervention. Bakhtin, a leading advocate of this approach, has suggested that each word in a narrative "tastes of the content and contexts in which it has lived its socially charged life ..." so that eventually it becomes part of a social dialogue (cf. Casey 1993, 26).

Recovering alternative and unexamined knowledge, not recognized in more conventional approaches, forms the *sine qua non* of stories. In this regard, narrative accounts of displaced women present an epistemological challenge to feminist and medical anthropology, which have not been able to accommodate substantively the lived reality of non-Western women. Furthermore, the discipline's concern to give voice to marginalized women has not gone beyond recognizing "that cultures are differently practised outside their original geographical homes" (Ong 1995a, 366). Neither does there exist an epistemological space for non-Western women to engage in dialogue with mainstream feminist thought (Agnew 1996, Behar and Gordon 1995). In the context of this project I bring to the fore the narratives of displaced women. These women, I argue, bring to light the not-quite-articulated knowledge that exists in between systems by virtue of the fact that they have crossed territorial and social borders. Ong observes that anthropology needs to reflect on the post-colonial situations whereby we increasingly live inside, outside and through the East–West divisions (1995a, 368). She argues that examined lives bred on the borderlands between cultures represent new imaginations about gender, age and self-knowledge. Ordinary women telling their own stories "inter-nationally," to use Ong's phrase, should establish epistemological and methodological points of intervention into feminist and medical anthropology.

By paying close attention to context and the narrative text (content), I have endeavoured to create conversational space through reflexive listening and reading that renders the texts replicable. As Dorothy Smith has explained it, the iterability of these stories fosters actual social relations between the reader and the narrative texts— between reading, writing, speaking, hearing subjects (1999, 134). Active texts are enabling as they lift the words and the scenes from the text and give them life. The actualization of this narrative potential takes place through language, where the text can potentially enter into someone's course of action. Smith observes that "the language of the individual consciousness lies on the borderline between oneself and the other. The word in language is half someone else's (cf. Bakhtin, 136). Narratives perform a similar task. They create "a position of telling and listening."

Stories must have a home in a community of listeners for whom the story makes a claim that will be remembered. The challenge here is to listen to the voices in a manner that allow us to capture the lived reality of the speakers while simultaneously to understand the shaping of this reality by the dominant system. Ultimately the task at hand is to recognize these women as producers of knowledge. It is only at this level that we can speak "with them" (conversational mode) and not "for them" (appropriating mode). The topic of displacement and mental health has been chosen for its dialogical potential, the complexities of which are discussed throughout this book. Focus on dialogue does not overlook the workings of power that pose innumerable barriers and cause undue suffering (multi-faceted), a theme also highlighted throughout this book.

In sum, this book represents one attempt to show the potential of narratives and storytelling to bring to the fore a different understanding of mental health and displacement—an understanding that goes beyond the common biomedical and therapeutic rendering of this topic. At the centre of my study are ordinary narrators whose experiential knowledge and ideas on health and displacement are barely known by the wider society. In keeping with the spirit of this work, Iranian women are presented as authors of their own narratives of displacement, mental health and resettlement in Canada.

In Chapter 2, I lay the groundwork for this book using narrative texts from a storytelling session. Chapters 3 and 4 introduce the reader to two salient themes identified in the narratives: "What it is like to be displaced?" and "What is it like for a displaced person to look for work?" as seen through the eyes of two women, Sultan and Nadia, respectively. Chapters 5 and 6 concentrate on two "special" themes that capture the life course of an elderly woman and a caregiver, topics narrated by Zahra and Fatima, respectively. Each of these chapters examines individual women's narratives to identify the particular contexts in which their stories unfold. Women's own understandings of "mental health" and their experiences of displacement are considered, as are points of connection (which does not exclude ruptures) for dialogue with members of a "listening community." The key issue here is that each of the speakers has moved beyond the discrete realm of biomedicine to present larger worlds that highlight issues of justice and sociality.

In the concluding chapter, I situate these speakers' narratives within the reconstituted contexts that they present, and I discuss the epistemological significance and the practical import—visionary pragmatism, to use Hill Collin's (2000) words—of their life narratives at a time when mental health services continue to remain firmly entrenched within the biomedical system. Hopefully, by the time the readers have finished this work, they will have a clearer understanding of the knowledge base that women have presented through their respective narratives; they will be able to place the several quotations that began this introduction into their ideological and political contexts; they will be able to situate themselves in the debate and discussion on "mental health" and displacement, both of which are best understood as social suffering.

Notes

1 There are 88,200 individuals of Iranian origin in Canada according to 2001 census (biblionet@statcan.ca).

2 This term is used in inverted comas because through telling stories of their lives Iranian women reconfigured it to give it a non-medicalized focus.

3 This term is also used by Gelya Frank in her work *Venus on Wheels* (2000).

4 Although I do not speak Farsi, I have cultural links with Iran. We celebrate the Iranian New Year and follow some of the ritual practices that originated in Iran. Before commencing field research, I took several lessons in Farsi.

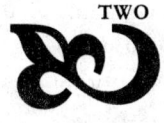

TWO

Authored and
Unauthored Texts

In 1905, the year preceding the Iranian Constitutional Revolution, the country was gripped by two events: the selling of daughters by distraught peasants, and the abduction of women and girls by Turkoman tribes. Both were related in the form of stories that were told and retold from the pulpits of the mosques, in political meetings and on the streets. Assuming the form of prose, poetry, satire and drama, the stories gripped the national imagination of Iran. This storied "event" forms the subject matter of Afsaneh Najmabadi's work, *The Story of the Daughters of Quchan*. She notes:

> Known as "Hikayat-i dukhataran-i Quchan" [the story of the daughters of Quchan], it was narrated in many forms and by diverse speakers and writers. Muslim preachers lamented the fate of the girls from the pulpit. Social Democratic militants used the story as a tale of the injustice of the rich and the tyranny of the rulers. The story was recited not only from the pulpit and in political leaflets. It worked as an exemplar in the burgeoning press, in a multiplicity of contexts, and through many literary forms: in dialogicals and letters of warning, in prose and poetry, in street songs and satire. (1998b, 1)

The nation focused on the women's captivity because the story's multiple retellings occurred at a time when Iran was undergoing political changes from autocratic rule towards a constitutional regime. What captured the attention of Najmabadi, an Iranian historian, and provided the rationale for writing and resurrecting this tale of grievance was the fact that after many retellings, this story eventually slipped into national amnesia. The women were used as ploys to advance patriarchal agendas. What was at stake was men's honour for failing to protect women; women's welfare was not the issue. Najmabadi then undertook the task of writing women into Iranian history on the grounds that their presence leads to narrating a different kind of history—one where the contradictory and contesting moments of women's everyday lives are valorized. Writing on another front, Farraneh Milani has chronicled one-and-a-half centuries of Iranian women's literary writings. Herself a poet and a literary scholar, she aims to capture women's struggles to counter their spatial and verbal exclusion from society and from the rich but male-oriented Iranian literature. Milani's project is informed by her own dilemma of having to address women's subordinate status in her home of Iran and adopted country of the United States. In the way of an example, she presents two images of the veil. The first is that of silence and immobility *(sokut-o-sokun)* that excludes women from the literary field (and other spheres of society); the second is the sense of security and certainty with which Milani grew up, despite living within the world of walls and veils. The author identifies an additional dimension of invisible veils and barriers that she encounters in her new home in United States. She writes:

> A poem ["Yasaman"] I wrote years ago best epitomizes my frantic search for bearings, for familiar boundaries. It portrays my internal turmoil at this point, as if I were running in two directions at once. One nostalgically backward for familiar walls and veils, for certainties lost, ... The other, frantically running sideways and forwards, to master the vertigo of open spaces, to master how to negotiate new, unfamiliar invisible walls ... (1992, xii)

As an immigrant, Milani finds herself writing in a foreign language about a group of female Iranian writers who have been exiled (marginalized) from their own land; a second level of exclusion arises from the fact that her literary works and those of other Iranian women are not recognized in the mainstream Anglo-American and world literature. She sees herself "as an exile writing about exiles" (Ibid., 13).

Najmabadi's and Milani's works represent a growing body of literature authored by Iranian women interested in seeing how women negotiate the aesthetics of silence and come to terms with gender and also racial "violence" and exclusion. Their second goal is to explore new territory and constitute new plots to see how women create art out of life: "the song of the mute and the dance of the immobile" (Milani 1992, xv).

Women's refusal to maintain silence and their attempts to explore new domains can occur at multiple levels and sites. One such level is that of ordinary immigrant women telling their stories in a foreign land. But these stories are markedly different from those of female literary writers whose work gets published. To begin with, these unauthored texts are grounded in everyday experiences, which are informed by larger socio-political forces that exclude and marginalize women in the first place. The important issue here is that these stories name and identify such forces while simultaneously creating spaces in which they can eventually become part of the national and the social landscapes of the society in question.

In this chapter, I explore the pedagogical potential of the stories of post-revolution Iranian women living in metropolitan Vancouver.[1] Our point of entry into the lives of these women is emotional well-being, a subject that is of interest for two reasons. First, among the many lenses deployed by dominant society to construct immigrant and refugee women as the Other, that of emotional well-being (mental health) is salient. Female newcomers are at a greater disadvantage than their male counterparts and European migrants. The dominant society and its institutions erroneously trace the source of their disadvantaged status to the cultures of these women's home countries—a strategy that masks structural factors of exclusion and racism (Agnew 1996, Bannerji 1995, Jiwani 2001, Razack 1998, Thobani 1999). Second, using the medium of stories, female newcomers frame the issue of emotional well-being differently than does the medical model, and in doing so they highlight broader and more inclusive parameters, as is evident from the fact that the participants in our study chose to use the term *emotional well-being* (read: wellness) as opposed to *mental health* (read: illness). Women's framing of emotional well-being in the way of a critique of the host society as well as their chalking of new paths must be contextualized—that is, considered in terms of the broader picture where social and economic forces are salient—so as to avoid a situation where their stories are appropriated rather than valorized.

Immigrant and refugee women's stories are appropriated and homogenized differently depending on the particular vantage point. For service providers (including the media), these women are fleeing from "an unremittingly oppressive society into full emancipation in the West" (Ong 1995a). If they have not been able to achieve a sense of freedom, so the conversation goes, they have to work harder and give themselves more time. In the eyes of the policy makers and prospective employers, these women's life experiences are of little consequence in the host country and hence they are being erased by the dominant system. Historical and ethnographic works that attempt to provide more nuanced profiles do not make their way into the corridors of power where decisions are made and policies formulated. One term that captures the above perceptions is *negative homogenization*.

In an attempt to reverse this trend, we will engage in "generous contextualization," to use the term suggested by Razack (1998, also see Farmer 2003). Adding contexts to women's stories leads to a paradigm shift from victim-blaming to unmasking the system's complicity in oppressing women. Analytical frameworks for deconstructing the system's operation at particular sites (courts, classrooms and workplace) have been well developed by feminist scholars in the developing world (Razack 1998, Bannerji). Citing the case of sexual and racist harassment of a Black woman in a Canadian workplace, Bannerji notes that this woman's experiences may best be understood in the context of her social location and work setting. More layered contexts, Bannerji argues, bring to light the fact that the workplace is not only a unit of economic production but a site "which is organized through known and predictable social relations, practices, cultural norms and expectations" (1995, 130). A reading of these relations of ruling, embedded in the Canadian history of colonization, leads Bannerji to conclude that social forces inform the Black woman's experience of harassment.

Structural analysis of sites where racialized women work and live have offered invaluable insights into their everyday experiences of racist and sexist oppression. But these frameworks do not leave much room for women to be seen as social actors and producers of knowledge, of value to the society in which they live. If their ideas are at all recognized they are confined to discrete and socially confined spheres (Moore 1996).

Keeping in mind the above focus, I have organized this chapter as follows. In the first part, I provide a profile of the veil as a point of intervention into the homogenized equation: veil = oppression. This discussion provides background information on Iranian storytellers[2] who related their pre- and post-migration experiences at a "women and well-being" session. In the second part, I present two more contexts—the political economy of health and critical pedagogy—to lay the groundwork for listening to the stories. These contexts pave the way for the third part, in which we will "read"[3] Iranian women's *(Zan-e Irani)* stories as part of a literary movement through which these women, at home and abroad, have begun to tell their tales loud and clear (Afkhami and Friedl 1994, Milani 1992). The conclusion examines the implications of storytelling for social change.

The Trajectory of the Veil
ൠ

During her lifetime, any elderly Iranian immigrant woman will have been subject to four behavioural phases related to the veil: traditional veiling from the time of puberty; forceful unveiling following the Shah's 1936 decree; forced re-veiling in the post-revolutionary era; and "invisible veiling and walls" in her adopted country of Canada. This observation raises one point: women's lives are embedded in history and in the social and economic conditions of the times, but not along a linear path. Veiled, unveiled or re-veiled, women respond to conditions that shape their lives and in the process suggest alternative ways of being. This commonplace knowledge needs to be reiterated because women may also find themselves in situations where they are rendered socially invisible and their life experiences are not validated or are dismissed as being inconsequential by the larger society.

✂ The Story of the Veil

Traditional veiling of women in Iran and elsewhere in the Middle East has been the subject of numerous works, many of which have been authored by Middle East women scholars (Ahmed 1992; Milani 1992; Mernissi 1975, 1991; Alvi et al. 2003). These works highlight nuanced historic and socio-specific contexts; the essential idea is to show that veiling in itself does not translate into seclusion or a subordinate position. Rather, it is the larger social, economic and ideological factors that determine women's social status.

Taking a historical perspective, Ahmed (1992) argues that women's veiling and segregation must be understood in the context of the tension between the legalistic politicized version of Islam and the ethical egalitarian approach embedded in the Qura'n. Anthropologist Erika Friedl offers a different perspective in her work over a period of two decades in an Iranian village. She notes that veiled women once were in a position to negotiate their presence in the male public world; however, this possibility has been minimized in the capitalistic market world, which has undermined women's networks and rendered them powerless. Her insights on women's "traditional" world are revealing: " ... locally women are said to belong in the house, yet one sees many women out on apparently legitimate errands, often all day and far from home. A respectable woman will argue that she cannot walk even a few steps down the lane to visit a relative without being wrapped in a long veil, yet the same woman can be seen working at the public water channel, not only sans cumbersome veil but with her shirt sleeves rolled up to her elbows" (1989, 196).

The Shah's 1936 decree of forced unveiling was politically motivated. Like other male "reformers" of the time, he believed that the modernization of Iran could not take place without using women as markers of national identity. In a modernized country, women must be (ostensibly) seen as liberated and taking their place alongside men. But in actual fact, only a few urban women were recipients of the "benefits" accruing from the modern projects of education and the market economy. The Shah's second goal was directed outwards. He wanted to project a particular image for the West, whose modernization model he had adopted unreservedly—

the equation being that Iran was progressive because its women were unveiled. But state-imposed changes are ambiguous. As Sullivan reminds us: "Life makes for strange bedfellows. Just as Big Oil, the United States and the Shah had no intention of producing an Islamic Revolution, so too the Islamic Revolution had no intention of producing its unintended effect: a potential that, though compromised, is realizing itself in a kind of women's movement specific to and produced by its historical movement ..." (1998, 236).

Thus women appropriated the state's rhetoric of female emancipation and worked towards improving the conditions of their lives. "For the first time in their history, Iranian women found their way into the parliament, the cabinet, the armed forces, the legal profession, and a variety of fields in science and high technology" (Afkhami and Friedl 1994, 11). It was women's lobbying that led to the introduction of the Family Protection Law (1976), giving Iranian women the right to decide, among other things, on matters of marriage, divorce and custody of children.

In post-revolution Iran, women are re-veiled by law. The Family Protection Law was repealed and the new regime introduced measures that tried "to force women out of the job market in a variety of ways, including early retirement of government women employees, closing of child-care centres, segregating women and enforcing full Islamic cover *(hejab-e islami)* in offices and public places, and closing nearly 140 university fields of study to women" (Ibid., 12). Yet women continued to fight for their rights and their struggles to some extent were bolstered by social and economic conditions. For example, the moderate gains that women made over five decades under the Shah's regime have not been completely erased.

Afkhami and Friedl note, first, that some of the rights that women achieved have settled into the collective psyche of the society. Second, the downward trend in Iran's post-revolution economy has made it necessary for women to stay in the job market. Third, the repealed Family Protection Law was replaced by contractual Islamic law under which marriage is considered to be an agreement between two individuals; here women now have some leeway to negotiate more favourable conditions such as "the condition of monogamy, the right of the woman to divorce, and the equitable division of the wealth accumulated during marriage. In general these conditions are more favourable to women than was the old Family Protection Law" (Moghadam 1994, 95). Despite constraints such as the absence of a legal requirement for husbands to make the contract egalitarian, the contract is popular, as attested by the fact that notary public offices have printed advanced copies of this document (Ibid., 95). Fourth, Iranian women's presence is felt in the arts, in literature, in cinema, in education and in politics. Even if the goals of freedom and equality evade them, as is also the case with many women in the West, women in Iran have created an atmosphere whereby their concerns have moved from the margins into the centre of Iranian society. And these accomplishments have been the result of the work of "veiled" women.

A caveat is in order. The above discussion does not assume that in Iran gender is a master status informing the lives of women. The discrepancy between rich and poor woman, and between rural and urban women, is pronounced. It is common knowledge that women's access to education and resources is shaped by their socioeconomic status. While not underplaying these and other differences such as ethnicity and religion, women's issues are at the forefront of the social, religious, economic and political life of the country. And as has been the case for centuries, these issues are debated by women themselves from their different social locations. Both in the way women have made moderate gains and in terms of their ongoing struggles for equality, they form part of the growing force for change within Iran. We now turn to the migrants who came to Canada in the post-revolution period.

❧ Invisible Veils/Walls

The structural location of post-revolution Iranian immigrant women in Canada is no different from that of other racialized women. Discursively constructed as the "Other" and subject to racism and sexism, these women have little opportunity to realize the promise of gender and race-based equality enshrined in the Canadian Charter of Rights. Racism is a lethal weapon used for continuous ghettoization and marginalization of immigrant women. The impact of this destructive force has been noted at various levels (Bannerji 2000). Inherently, racism is a mode of exclusion, subordination and exploitation that operates in different forms governed by specific historical and social contexts. Entrenched in systems and institutions, it operates in multiple ways along the same lines as Foucault's (1973, 1978) model of power in modern societies.

Dua (1999), Thobani (1999), Jiwani (2001), Mohanty (2003) and Ng (1988/1996) have differentially noted the deficiency discourse that surrounds the [socially constructed category of an immigrant woman from the developing world: she does not speak English; she is passive, oppressed, and home-bound; she is usually found in the lower echelons of the workforce; and, if labeled a refugee, she is a drain on the system.] The structural location of immigrant women is that of subordination. "Their inequality is defined on the basis of economic, socio-cultural and political devaluation, all of which are underpinned by historical and contemporary social forces and institutionalized in society" (Jiwani 2001, 5). An additional factor that defines the situation of Muslim women in the West is the veil.

In the Western world, the veil is not viewed as a piece of attire with a complex trajectory, as illustrated above with reference to the Iranian situation. Rather, the meaning ascribed to the veil is tied to the colonial narrative of the oppression of Muslim women, the historical context of which is outlined in Leila Ahmed's (1992) work, *Women and Gender in Islam*. Ahmed argues that the West's use of the veil as a symbol of oppression served two purposes. First it established the West's superior status over the colonized Muslim world based on the argument that Muslim societies' oppression of women was the outcome of their barbaric culture and religion, which needed to be replaced by the West's civilizing mission. Second, the colonial narrative served to appropriate feminist discourse at home and channelled it to the East ("white men saving brown women from brown men," as Spivak [1988] has expressed it). The idea is to undermine Western feminism, an approach that white feminists unfortunately adopted to their own disadvantage; along with their male counterparts, white women positioned themselves to save brown women from the clutches of what they perceived as the oppressive culture of the colonized. Ahmed reiterates this point: "European feminists critical of the practices and beliefs of the men of their societies with respect to themselves acquiesced in and indeed promoted the European male's representations of Other men and the culture of Other men and joined in the name of feminism, in the

attack on the veil and the practices generally of Muslim societies"
(1992, 243).

The colonialist lens has followed Muslim women into their new
homeland in the West. The "oppression" of Muslim women is invoked
in the Western media, in the social service sector, and in scholarship
for the sole purpose of constructing these women in the image of
the alien Other (Hoodfar 1997). As Modood has observed in the
case of Europe, "Muslims are indeed very much a part of 'the
otherness' in the self-definition of the various peoples of the region"
(1997, 2). Under such forceful impulses the power of the colonial
narrative has not declined. Ahmed reminds us "that the measure of
whether Muslim women were liberated or not lay in whether they
veiled and whether the particular society had become 'progressive'
and Westernized or insisted on clinging to Arab and Islamic ways"
(1992, 247).

The social construction of the immigrant Muslim women as the
racialized Other constitutes the fourth phase of the trajectory in the
veil. But the veil in this context is not material; structurally, it has
assumed the form of invisible walls that block post-revolution
Iranian women's participation in Canadian society. The difference
between the first three phases of the trajectory of the veil (its story)
and the last is as follows. In the first three phases, conditions and
spaces existed for women to work towards improving their life
situations, despite multiple experiences of reversal. In the fourth
phase, it is the non-existence of these conditions that is the issue,
and it is at this fundamental level that the well-being of Iranian
women in Canada has been affected.

Invisible Veils/Walls and Emotional Well-being
&

The correlation between visible veiling/unveiling, invisible veiling/
walls, and emotional well-being may be explained along the following
lines. To begin with, both visible and invisible veiling have prevented
women from developing their potential for full participation in
society. But there is a difference in kind between the two forms of
veiling. In Iran, despite living in a gender-segregated world with its

shaded history of gains and losses, Iranian women, as explained above, have had some space to negotiate the conditions of their lives. As Iranian and other Middle East female scholars have informed us, this is because women have had access to mediums of expression. Here are a few examples. Milani observes that over the last 150 years Iranian women have turned to poetry and prose "to free women's public voices" (1992, 1). Iranian women's literary tradition, she argues, has its roots in the age-old art of spinning tales. On another front, anthropologist Erika Friedl has observed the multiple and ingenious ways in which women negotiate the realities of their everyday lives. She notes that despite women's dependent position in society, "they use their culture, their relationships, and their philosophy to construct their lives and the lives of those near them" (1989, 6). Women's presence in the political and moral imagination of Iranian society is also revealed in publications such as *Zanan*, a monthly magazine that advocates gender equality.

On the Canadian scene, however, the kind of multiple media through which women continue to struggle for their rights in Iran are totally absent. Here, Iranian women (and men) may be noticed as recipients of services, as was the case with our cohort of research participants; their presence is acknowledged negatively through stereotypes. For example, within the social service sector, the two common phrases that I came across during my research were "They are illiterate," and "They are stupid."[4] It appears that these assumptions implicitly determined women's limited access to services. These negative perceptions have led to the creation of additional barriers in the form of invisible walls, which compound Iranian women's[5] social invisibility and, as noted above, essentially translate into erasure of their historical trajectories of struggle.

Two things have a particular impact on an individual's emotional well-being: the absence of social arenas that allow her to fight for her rights, and the absence of spheres of activities and relationships where her presence is acknowledged and her contributions are recognized. While this appears to be well known, the processes through which an individual's life experiences are erased are not easily understood. What are the circumstances that prompt the cohort of our research participants to say, "I am tired of life," "I have nothing to live for," "I get up in the morning feeling very sad and when I go back to bed, my sadness is there," and "I live with pain every day." These are strong statements, and their incorporation in the DSM-IV (Diagnostic and Statistical Manual) mapping of mental health would categorize these women as "patients" in need of therapy. But this is not the route the participants choose. As one woman explained it, "I am looking for a long-term solution. I am not going to go to the doctor and get antidepressants for my pain and suffering." Another woman related her friend's story to make the point that the medical solution undermined women's survival power—a power of which they were acutely aware despite ups and downs in their well-being:

> My friend has been very depressed. She continued to struggle. She had a list of six telephone numbers of her friends. She had memorized these numbers and she would call one friend at a time and talk to her at length. I was one of those friends. One day, her son insisted that she visit a doctor. The doctor prescribed antidepressants. She felt better for a few months but then her depression came back. This time the doctor gave her a stronger dose. Every time she went to him, he increased her dosage. You know what has happened to her? She has stopped calling her friends. The last time I saw her, she was numb. She did not want to talk. This is what medication does to you. It takes away your power to struggle.

Mainstream health institutions do not accept Iranian women's own understanding of emotional well-being—the existential understanding identified above. Here, if health care workers address the concerns of Iranian and other immigrant women at all, they do so as issues. Inaccessibility arising from language and "cultural" barriers receives primary importance, followed by recognition of social determinants of health, which may or may not include the impact of racism on women's lives (Morrow and Chappell 1999). There is equal emphasis placed on immigrant women's inability to integrate into the host society because, in the words of one service provider, "they are not equipped to live here." The factors cited are "inability to speak English" and "cultural oppression." For Muslim women an additional factor is her veil (read: she is backward and oppressed). An ESL teacher related that she had had a veiled woman in her class. She would not look in her direction, thinking the student was unintelligent. Not until halfway through the term, after the woman spoke, did it dawn on the teacher that the veiled woman was the brightest in her class.

A cursory glance indicates that the recommendations made in community reports on immigrant women (Canadian Task Force on Mental Health 1988; Morrow and Chappell 1999) follow a continuum: anti-racist strategies are placed at one end, and culturally sensitive issues are placed at the other end. The contradictions between the two are barely recognized: the former call for structural changes while the latter keep the structure intact. Also included are alternative family- and community-oriented systems of care practised by immigrant communities. Ultimately, the model of care (culturally sensitive or otherwise) is individualized: the onus of integrating into the host society and maintaining well-being is placed on women themselves. The individualized and politicized models denude the historical and social trajectories of women's lives.

Storytelling constitutes one avenue through which women's complex lives may be captured within a temporal framework: what the past was like, what the present ought to be, and how the future is envisioned.

Stories then require second and third readings, made possible through generous contextualization, for which purpose I have included the relevant literature in the body of the narrative texts. It is within these contextualized readings that we may begin to appreciate the story's potential for change, in that they challenge the us/them boundaries and question the validity of received knowledge. Inasmuch as they capture the world of people who have experienced pain and suffering, the stories of marginalized people are bound to suggest knowledge of a just world (Razack 1998, Dossa 2002).

The above discussion establishes one point: stories and narratives have the potential to effect social change provided they form part of the larger political, social, historical, cultural and literary landscapes of societies. Unfortunately, the possibility of Iranian and other immigrant women becoming part of the Canadian landscape is remote, as their structural and social exclusion is intense. Yet their stories must be heard if we want to write a different kind of Canadian history, one in which women from different cultural and linguistic backgrounds have an active presence. As Trinh has expressed it: "It will take a long time, but the story must be told" (1989, 119). In this spirit I present stories from the group session on emotional well-being.[6] It was evident that women who shared their stories were looking for avenues to change the conditions of their lives, if only in a small way.

Our listening, then, must be focused on the lives of those who tell their stories and what we do with the stories once we have heard them. Each story has its own point of entry. In the following section, I suggest an entry point from my home discipline of anthropology. I have paid close attention to moments, occurrences and words that might otherwise be dismissed as inconsequential; but at the same time, my engagement with the discipline has been informed by the need to address its unrealized goal of tacit humanism—a goal that has remained suspended owing to the discipline's historical complicity with the colonizing project.

Telling Their Stories on Emotional Well-being
∞

That a cohort of Iranian women[7] participated in the storytelling session did not give me the license to assume that there was automatic friendship, goodwill and a sense of togetherness within the group. Social hierarchies are present within subordinate groups, and to assume that the Iranian women's concerns were homogenous would have defeated the purpose of the session. Critical pedagogy cannot be built on unexamined assumptions such as the universal oppression of women. The challenge, then, is to examine the process of how women worked toward establishing a forum for expressing their concerns about emotional well-being. Two moments illustrate this point further: "Starting Points" and "Epitomizing Narratives."

∞ Starting Points

Ethical issues surrounding field research involving human participants have been addressed in the academy through letters of solicitation and consent forms. Accordingly, I distributed letters and forms in Farsi (Persian) and English to members of the group. Participants politely acknowledged my verbal explanation of the content of this material—for example, maintenance of confidentiality and the right of participants to refuse to take part in, or to withdraw from, the research. This top-down approach was substituted by the participants, who introduced their own practice: they took the oath of confidentiality verbally and through the gesture of raising the right hand.

Furthermore, participants' right to withdraw from the study was converted into its opposite: they decided that they would commit to attending all of the sessions. Ironically, trust and goodwill were fostered through subversion of the system (the ethics regulations and paperwork); it appears that the participants had an intuitive understanding that protection of individual rights does not contribute to group-building. This is in keeping with the liberal democratic model that emphasizes individual rights but does not advocate group rights. Charles Taylor's (1994) much-cited work on communitarian values has been critiqued by Bannerji on the grounds that it is an "elitist form of self-deception, which in the name of the community offers condescension" (2000, 149).

When I had first approached the Iranian coordinator, it was my expectation that she would select participants according to the research criteria I had given her: (1) age 33 to 66; (2) migration to Canada over the last fifteen years; and (3) both lower and upper class. During my conversation with the coordinator, I learned that these criteria were not used: "I have chosen the participants who represent the concerns of the 70 Iranian women who participate in the ESL programme." This point was confirmed by one of the participants in the class: "Our stories are everyone's stories." The Iranian women were keen to present a united front, knowing full well that this was one way in which they could make their stories known. Yet, the women wanted to ensure that I understood the significance of each of their stories, while not losing sight of a common landscape. An illustrative example comes from our introductions:

- We came to Canada two-and-a-half years ago. I have two sons, 13 and 8 years old. My husband is a medical practitioner; I am a clinical psychologist and am a certified dental assistant.
- I am married and I live with my husband. I have two grown-up children. I have been in Canada for eleven years.

- I live with my husband and I have six children. One son lives in America. Three of my children live with me. The rest are married. We have been in Canada for four years.
- I have two grown up children. My children do not live with me. I am here with my husband. I have been in Canada for ten years.
- I am a widow. I have three sons and two daughters. They are all grown up and married. I am alone and often sick. I have been in Canada for eight years.
- I have been in Canada for twenty-one years. I feel like an immigrant. I have been doing voluntary work for six years. I am a retired nurse (mainstream/white coordinator).
- I am an anthropologist from Simon Fraser University. I am doing research on the emotional well-being of Iranian women. I am originally from Uganda and I have been in Canada for thirty years (researcher).

Introductions are usually glossed over, as they are considered to be a warm-up exercise to facilitate discussion of more substantive issues. For the participants in our study, however, introductions, as well as the research criteria and other strategies we examined above, may be considered a framing device. They allow the women to establish parameters before commencing the work of telling their stories.

There are two entry points in the introductions. The first one concerns motherhood. My initial reading of the texts led me to conclude that the women chose this particular entry point because they considered the role of motherhood critically important. As elsewhere in the world, motherhood is also a social construct that brings to the fore dilemmas and tensions: for example, home versus career life, the "de-skilling process" that their work has been subjected to globally (Mohanty 2003, Harrison 1997), and medicalization of their bodies, especially during critical periods such as birthing and aging (Ram and Jolly 1998, Lock 1993). A second reading of the introduction suggests that women were putting forward an agenda—to raise the issue of the tension-filled role of motherhood that mainstream women do not discuss often in the public sphere. (Consider the very different introductions of the mainstream coordinator and the researcher included above.)

In choosing to foreground their role as mothers, Iranian women established a different point of entry that undermined the private versus public divide and created a broader expanse within which they could relate their stores of emotional well-being. Yet, the participants did not gloss over their different experiences of motherhood. The introductions reveal different vantage points: a young mother with three occupations, mothers who lived with or away from their children, and a widow. These vantage points made space for women to relate their different experiences without losing sight of their common concerns as people in search of meaningful engagement with life in their country of adoption.

In their introductions participants also commented on the number of years they had been in Canada. The mention of the time period may be in response to service providers' common assumption that the longer the newcomers are in Canada, the greater is their level of integration. This widely held notion places the onus on the individual "to settle down," diverting attention from issues of racism and structural barriers. In presenting the different time frames: two-and-a-half years to eleven years, the participants are giving the message that the period of residence and integration cannot be conflated. The "starting points" included another element: the "naming" of emotional well-being—that is, giving the term their own meaning. The entry point here is that the participants had been exposed to and had knowledge of the dominant mental-health discourse. Through attending orientation sessions of service programmes and sharing stories such as the one cited above (depression = medication = numbness), the women identified two issues: first, inaccessibility of services owing to linguistic and material constraints, and second, inappropriateness of the term *mental health*.

During the initial phase of my research, the participants suggested that I not use the term *mental health*. "It means being crazy," said one woman. They recommended that I use the term *emotional well-being*. They also rejected the Iranian term *narahati*, which connotes "undifferentiated unpleasant emotional and physical feelings" (Pliskin 1987, 47; Good 1977). In his work on Iranian immigrants in Israel, Pliskin notes that *narahati* refers to "a wide range of negative emotions, some of which were explained to me by Iranians in Israel as depressed, inconvenienced, nervous, anxious, troubled, uneasy, worried, upset, disappointed, bothered, not tranquil, being in a bad mood, not feeling well, restless" (Ibid., 47). This definition, confirmed by two physicians, a psychologist and two service providers (all Iranians) nests within the biomedical model: it focuses exclusively on the issue of illness and it is depoliticized. Exercising intuitive immediacy[8] (a pragmatic as well as an in-depth understanding of the issues), the participants suggested that we use the term *Salamat-e Ruh* instead. *Salamat* means "peace" and *Ruh* is translated as "soul."

Of interest is the fact that the participants were bent on conveying only one message: disruption of a person's state of peace and the impact on a person's soul are serious matters and should not be dismissed lightly. They conveyed this message through stories, examples of which are discussed below in the form of epitomizing moments. In opting to use the term *Salamat-e Ruh*, the participants were drawing our attention to the existential dimension of living— the terms peace and soul cannot be located at a superficial level as they touch on the very being of a person. Disruption of *Salamat-e Ruh* evokes an intense struggle to maintain one's well-being. The form of "struggle" that I refer to here is markedly different from the host society's understanding of struggle, as expressed in this way: "It is all right if they have to take low-pay work even if they were professionals back at home. All immigrants who come to Canada struggle" (field notes, March 2000). For Iranian women the struggle in question involves engaging meaningfully with life situations in their adopted country—a theme highlighted in the women's stories. The meaning of *Salamet-e Ruh* may be understood at this fundamental level.

Critical pedagogy requires us to pay close attention to the ground-clearing activity that the speakers engage in to create a new and more expanded space where they can tell the stories of their lives without having to use the parameters of dominant society. With this in mind I have included the participants' starting points, or the framing activity.

In the above section, I have attempted to show that in creating an expanded space (as opposed to the confined parameters of the medical model of mental health), the participants have located themselves to tell two intertwined stories: those of their own lives, and those of the dominant society's exclusionary practices. They raised the issue of emotional well-being as expressed through the medium of *Salamat-e Ruh*. The stories bring to light the pain as well as the survival power of women, the telling of which may best be captured at particular epitomizing moments in their stories. This moment in question is a women's (W) conversation with a representative (R) of the dominant system.[9]

W: Why can I not get work in Canada?

R: You can't find work because you do not know our language?

W: I am not sure, whether this is correct. I have taken English in school and I am taking lessons here. If I am given the opportunity, I can learn quickly.

R: It is up to you. You first learn the language before you can even expect to find work. Do you speak English at home?

W: How can I do this? It is my responsibility to make sure that my children learn Farsi. Home is the only place where they can do this.

R: Well, it is up to you. You have to make hard choices in a new country.

W: My friend speaks very good English. How come she cannot find work?

R: Well, it is because she does not have the Canadian experience.

W: How can she get Canadian experience when no one hires her?

R: Ask her to do voluntary work.

W: Voluntary work can take years and years but it does not help us to get a job.

R: You have to work harder. Other immigrants have made it and you will too.

W: How about you listening to my story. It says all. I cannot tell the whole story, it is too painful. Do you have a moment to listen to our stories?[10]

❧ Epitomizing Narratives

Epitomizing narratives refer to situations that highlight the impact of socio-economic factors as well as human agency. This perspective, which is embedded in the act of storytelling and for which I have made a contextualized case above, will guide my reading of the following stories.[11]

Sahra, a journalist by profession, spoke first. She said that she was a good listener and therefore a lot of women had confided their life stories to her. She expressed her desire to share a sad story that was the story of "every Iranian woman." After uttering one sentence, however, tears rolled down her cheeks and she said: "I cannot continue. It is too painful."

The storytelling session began on the note of silence. But this gesture must not be dismissed as of no consequence. Anthropologist Visweswaran suggests that "we should be attentive to silence as a marker of women's agency"; women's refusal to speak should make us investigate when and why women do talk (1994, 51). The intensity of Sahra's pain could not be put into words but it alerts us to another medium of communication that may also include the element of paradox, as Susan Gal, also an anthropologist, has argued. Silence can be both a symbol of passivity and powerlessness as well as a form of political protest. In the latter case, one's refusal to speak is a strategic defense against the powerful (1991,175).

Sahra's silence incorporates an additional dimension of testimonio, "concerned not so much with the life of a 'problematic hero' ... as with the problematic collective social situation in which the narrator lives" (Beverley 1992, 95). We may note, that the participants'[12] efforts to present a front of solidarity takes place at the more intricate level of silence—a strategy made possible through the groundwork laid at the beginning of the session: Starting Points. Sahra's unspoken story is taken up by a second narrator, Simin. Simin began her story on the note of *Salamat-e Ruh*. She said that her state of well-being has been affected by two things: separation from her children and her not being able to work in Canada.

Simin is a mother of four children, three of whom live in the United States and one in Germany. This situation is painful for her, as in her words: "I am all alone with my husband." But she did not plan it this way. The sole reason why she left Iran was this: "There is nothing left in Iran for me. My children came to Canada and so I joined them." Her children went where the jobs were—a step they were compelled to take as there was no work for them in Canada despite the fact that they are all professionals. Simin said that it was a long and difficult process for her to get landed immigrant status and she did not want to go through the same cycle to join her children in yet another foreign country. This is because, as Thobani (1999) has shown, women's applications are processed through the family class of dependency in contrast to the independent class through which men's are processed. Women's secondary status translates into a slower and more arduous process; hence Simin's reluctance to go through this process a second time.

A second factor at work is the market economic model. Rooted in colonial capitalism, this model shortchanges racialized minorities, people in the non-Western world and most severely the women (Harrison 1997, Tinker 1997). Hierarchical structuring of labour compounds this situation: the market economic model requires the labour of younger and educated individuals; aging women, especially racialized women, fall by the wayside (Dossa 1999). Simin explained that her separation from the children would not be so painful if she was gainfully occupied. She desires the opportunity to learn English and work in her area of expertise, as a hairdresser and, beyond that, an advocate of women's rights. But none of these are within her reach and it is this void—"when I get up in the morning, I have nothing to look forward to"—that she identifies as the source of disruption of *Salamat-e Ruh*. It is at this juncture that she tells her story of what work meant to her in Iran and how lack of meaningful work is undermining her sense of well--being.

Simin presents herself as a very active woman:

> I was the executive director of a hairdressing salon and beauty salon. I was called upon to act as an examiner of hairdressing graduates. As the director of [a] women's association, I sat in the parliament. My work made it necessary for me to travel. I was very very busy. I have a lot of pictures of myself. My sister, she stayed at home and cooked *ghormeh sabji* [an Iranian delicacy]. I very much regret that I do not know English. I could have continued to work as a hairdresser. I can tell what colour of hair would be suitable for each person and what style would suit her best. Now I feel nobody. My life is useless. I feel tired.

At this point, we may make one observation: Simin gives a relatively longer account of her life accomplishments compared with her "symptoms" of a disrupted state of well-being. This is because

Simin's interest in telling her story is to emphasize one point: the importance of being meaningfully occupied. Simin conveys the message that her accomplishments have not occurred as a matter of course. She compares her life with that of her sister (her only sibling) who decided to cook *ghormeh sabji*—meaning she decided to stay at home. *Ghormeh sabji* is made of finely chopped vegetables, meat and beans and takes many hours to prepare; it is specially cooked for guests underpinning which is the idea of cultivating social ties. In bringing into sharper relief her public life, Simin does not denigrate her sister's domestic work.

By providing details of her work such as acting as an examiner, travelling and having her pictures taken—activities that she said she undertook voluntarily to advance women's causes—she brings to light the fact that these are special accomplishments for a woman whose domestic responsibilities are equally demanding. She related that she would stay up late at night to take care of housework. Farrokhzad[12](cf. Milani 1992) captures the agony of Iranian women compelled to choose between "careers" and motherhood:

> Every morning from behind the bars
> My child's eyes smile at me
> As I begin happily to sing,
> His kissing lips near mine.
> O God! If I need to fly out one day
> From behind those lonesome bars
> How will I answer this child's crying eyes?
> Let me be, a captive bird am I.

In these stanzas, Farrokhzad lays out the issues facing a woman who aspires to have career and be a mother. If she does not pay attention to her vocational aspirations, she deprives herself of the opportunity to be someone in the public world; but if she pursues her career, she is unable to fulfill societal expectations where a woman is no more than a daughter, a sister, a wife or a mother. In Simin's case, migration has meant a loss of not only a hard-built career but her accomplishment of building a bridge—however fragile—between two worlds that are incompatible for women.

The crucial point made in Simin's story is that the very ground on which women struggled to meet the competing demands of work and home life is no longer in place. In Canada, "there is nothing for me to do," she explained. It is at this fundamental level—the non-existence of opportunities to set and reach goals—that she grounds her state of *Salamat-e Ruh*.

Salamat-e Ruh is a term that first and foremost suggests the idea of well-being. Its corollary *salaam* (peace) is used in everyday greetings within Iran and the Islamic world. Recognition of its state of disruption points to the fact that one's being is affected at its core. But when one's core is affected negatively, one's survival power is activated. Simin is quick to point out her ways of coping with the situation: "I talk to myself, I talk to my friends and I talk to God." She stated that what keeps her going is the idea of visiting her children. "The thought that I would be visiting my children in United States or my son in Germany is important to me." She continued: "Many times, I look at the pictures and think about my life—how filled it was with meaning." This form of reconstruction of meaning is the focus of Gay Becker's (1997) work *Disrupted Lives: How People Create Meaning in a Chaotic World*. Becker's research participants engage in discursive reality, considered a form of self-healing. But Simin went further and related a practical step that she has undertaken in the hope that it would free her from feeling suffocated from isolation and loneliness. She is registered in an English language programme:

> I was determined to learn English. I registered myself in what I thought was a good programme. I soon realized that the programme would not work for me. I noticed that the teacher was discriminating. For her there were two kinds of students: those who were rich and those who were on welfare. She [the teacher] identified the rich ones through their tape recorders and $50 dictionaries. The teacher did not pay much attention to me and she was going very fast. I would go to class, open my book and at the end of the day close it without writing anything. I almost had a nervous breakdown. I could not go to classes for two weeks.
>
> When I went back, it was just before Christmas. I took a gift for the teacher. She accepted my gift. At the end of the day she told

me that I could no longer come to class as I had missed too much.
The actual reason was that they had found another rich student.

Reflecting on this experience, Simin related: "This incident happened four and a half years ago. Four and a half years have passed and now, if I were to start again, my capacity to learn is less." She suggested that her life could have been a little different: "If I had the opportunity to learn English, I would not have to look for people who can telephone for me to find out why I had not received credit from the hydro company." (She refers to the B.C. Hydro rebate given to consumers in British Columbia in January 2001.)

Simin's relation of details brings into relief the contours of the everyday world that in the case of marginalized people need to be problematized to reveal the operation of a whole range of soico-economic forces (Bannerji 1995, 131).

Simin highlighted language and work in her story. Framing these two issues in the form of a story, as opposed to making mere statements, brings home the lived reality of people whose life situations are subject to erasure upon migration. Simin does not say "I am a hairdresser," the sentence that she would be compelled to use if she was sitting in front of an employment counselor—perhaps an immigrant women's agency as shown in the work of Roxana Ng (1996). Here her credentials would most likely be converted into a dead-end job and more recently into dead-end volunteer work required in the cash-strapped service sector. "I have worked hard all my life and I have always been an active woman," says Simin as she nears the end of her story.

It is evident that Simin has established a clear focus around which she frames her story. Her sole purpose is to contrast her work in Iran, around which she had built her life, with the lack of opportunities for any kind of gainful employment (including non-waged work) in Canada. Simin is well aware of her linguistic "limitations," which she tries to correct to no avail. Although she starts her narrative with two "things that bother me," separation from children and not being able to work in Canada, it is the latter aspect that she addresses more vehemently. Perhaps this is the area where she thinks she has greater control. "I want to do something with my life. I am looking for a long-term solution" were the words that echoed at various points in her story. Also, she knows that this is an area of concern to her peers, who, in their own narratives, take her story further.

Nuri, a younger woman, began her story by categorically stating that she has three professions: "I am a clinical psychologist, a dental hygienist as well as a computer typist." She then explained that she had updated her language skills in Canada and "yet, I am not getting a job. I tried everywhere and there is no place for me. My husband is a medical practitioner. He took his board exams and is fluent in English. After sending 100 applications, he found part-time (two days a week) job in a medical clinic. Myself, I am doing volunteer work in hospitals and schools." Responding to a question on the possible value of voluntary work for learning English, she said: "No. I have no opportunity to learn the language. I work with senile elderly people or very small children." Nuri then recalled how one service provider had suggested that she should do volunteer work at a daycare centre. The service provider told her, "Don't worry if you think your English is not good. You can hold babies."

Nuri's story is intense, with a single focus that subverts the dominant society's framing of job opportunities for Iranian women: they cannot find work because they cannot speak English. By emphasizing her three qualifications and her husband's profession, upgraded to meet the Canadian requirements, Nuri strategically positions herself to speak with authority. Her discussion of her volunteer position brings home the structural vulnerability of racialized women. It is primarily women who are channelled into an exploitative voluntary sector that has emerged as a result of the state's downsizing of the service sector (Lee 1999). Of interest is the fact that Nuri leaves it to the reader to further interpret the service provider's suggestion: "Don't worry if you think your English is not good. You can hold babies." Nuri's decision not to elaborate on this further—whether she responded to or followed the service provider's suggestion—and maintain silence can be explained with reference to Gumperz's observation that the use of speech and silence "are strategic actions, created in responses to cultural and institutional contexts" (cf. Gal 1991,176). The institutional and cultural contexts are well laid out by Bannerji (1995), who states that Canada's ethnicized immigration history has governed hierarchical organization of the workplace on the grounds of "race," gender and class. Racialized women are normatively expected to hold dead-end and low-paid jobs. When the latter are not available, these women end up having no jobs, as was the case with Nuri. But Nuri is not a passive observer. Her narrative strategy of focusing on a particular issue with an endnote of silence evokes responses from other women in the group.

The fourth speaker related her story of secondary migration. She had lived in Sweden for five years before coming to Canada. While in Sweden she learned the language and then trained and worked as a cook. "In Canada, no one would hire me. One day I went to a Swedish reception. I met someone there who offered me a job in his restaurant. Is it not strange that in Canada, it is people from another country who gave me a job?"

The preceding story contains a paradox: the foreign country taking on the responsibility of giving her a job denied to her by her country of adoption. As she expressed it: "It is like your guest taking care of a family member." She found this paradox intriguing because "I came to Canada as a landed immigrant. My application was accepted just because I am a cook. I was told at the embassy that cooks are required in Canada."

A fifth speaker related a generational story. She began with the words "Everyone is saying that things will be better for our children. We have to struggle so that our children will have a better life. But listen to the story of my daughter." This woman then explained that her daughter had a hard time during the Iranian revolution. "To heal her spirit, she turned to Sufism (Islamic mysticism) and decided to wear the veil. She went to school in Canada and her first job was at the restaurant. They gave her kitchen work for only one reason: she wears the veil." This story is a poignant reminder of the structural vulnerability of Iranian women in Canada.

In their own ways, each speaker subverts the dominant dysfunctional discourse on immigrant women: they cannot work (except in the lower echelons of the labour market) because they do not have the right qualifications.

Iranian women's stories in Canada are told at a time when their counterparts in Iran are raising their voices and telling their tales through film, writing and other modes available to them. "Even those who portray themselves as victims of society—conforming, enduring, suffering—are gaining a significant victory in being able to plead their own cases and make their stories heard in their own words. They are survivors, the ultimate rebels, irrepressible, vocal, and articulate" (Milani 1992, 234).

Conclusion: Producing Knowledge through Storytelling

ও৲

In this chapter, I have provided generous contextualization of these women's stories. Based on the metaphors of "the veil" and "invisible walls," the context delineated is that of racialization of immigrant Iranian women, a situation that impacts on their state of well-being. I have argued that Iranian women's well-being must be addressed in relation to the dominant discourse of pathology where the onus is placed on the women themselves: they cannot find work because they do not have the qualifications; a second script is that of culture. It is these factors, so the argument goes, that affect women's mental health in a negative way. More recent work has begun to identify issues of racism together with the need for the delivery of more inclusive health services (for example, Anderson 1996; Dyck 1998)). But the suggested strategies remain locked within the biomedical model of care that does not address structural and social issues, not to mention the fact that the model is one of "illness" rather than a "wellness."

Iranian participants in our study had an intuitive understanding of these issues. In their stories, they did not discuss their experiences of *naharati* (depression). Yet, the majority of the participants acknowledged that their doctors had treated them medically for depression. The period of depression identified ranged from three months to one year, with the exception of one woman who said that she was chronically depressed. Diagnosis and therapy were not the topics that the participants dwelled on; some of the women talked about coping strategies grounded in everyday life activities.

Iranian women's stories are premised on the model of wellness. In framing their stories around this term, the women established a different terrain—one that included fundamental issues that the reader or listener can attend to. The issues at stake were those of entitlements: every human being has the right to work and be meaningfully occupied in her day-to-day life. The participants made this point by telling stories of what life was like in the past (in Iran), what the present is or ought to be like, and what the future could hold for them. The latter the women posed as a question, since their future—the way they envisioned it—did not seem attainable. Through ground-clearing activity, initiated by the women (the starting points), and the telling of epitomizing narratives (highlighting structure and agency), the women created space to tell their stories in a manner that should evoke the attention of the researcher/reader/ listener.

Within the limited scope of this chapter, the point that I have highlighted is that the issue of emotional well-being (mental health, in the dominant parlance) does not exclusively belong to the clinics, nor can it be framed as "social determinants of health"; the latter is of immense value in broadening the parameters of biomedicine, but its laundry-list format can only lead to fragmentary solutions.

Through storytelling, the women have gently directed the issue of emotional well-being to where it belongs: at the multiple sites where people live, work, learn and socially interact. It is logical to assume that knowledge on health, well-being and other concerns that we share as human beings should be produced in spaces of social interaction. This understanding, embedded in the stories I have included here, have been lost in the corridors of power (policy makers, funding agencies, the state's infrastructure) where decisions are made away from people's experiential knowledge of health and life. Storytelling is one medium through which the process of retrieval of knowledge, in the way of fresh perspectives and alternative insights, can begin. This is not a new argument. Anthropologists have long recognized that talk and narrative/storied conversations across cultures can lead to the construction of a more humane and inclusive knowledge base. This has yet to be realized.

Notes

1   I encouraged women to tell the stories of their lives. I consider this to be the best way to glean women's own understanding of emotional well-being—a term suggested by the participants.

2   I use this term in the generic sense. Iranian women are known to be skilled at the art of spinning tales (Milani 1992).

3   The emphasis is on critical reading, the groundwork for which is laid out in the contexts that Iranian woman highlighted in their stories.

4   Although these terms were not used by all service providers, they informed their attitudes and behaviour towards Iranian women in relation to particular contexts.

5   I would like to remind the reader that my usage of the term *Iranian women* only includes the cohort of women who participated in the study. I make no attempt to generalize their situation to other Iranian women living in metropolitan Vancouver.

6   This session was held concurrently with ESL classes.

7   The participants were six Iranian women, one mainstream coordinator, one Iranian coordinator-translator and myself.

8   Iranian anthropologist Erika Friedl (1989) argues that this is an important issue for women who are otherwise rendered socially invisible.

9   I have reconstructed this recurring conversation from my field notes.

10 Emphasis on cost-effectiveness in the delivery of services has minimized the time that service providers spend in listening to what the women have to say, let alone their stories.

11 To break the monotony of using one term, I have used *Iranian women, speakers, storytellers* and *participants* interchangeably.

12 Although Farrokhzad wrote in the early part of the 20th century, the concerns that she articulates are relevant today for women in the North and the South.

THREE

Being a Refugee in Canada:
Sultan's Story

"Asylum states and international agencies dealing with refugees, as well as much of the policy-oriented, therapeutic literature on refugees, tend to share the premise that refugees are essentially 'a problem.' Not just 'ordinary people,' they are constituted, rather, as an anomaly requiring specialized correctives and therapeutic interventions." (Malkki 1995, 8)

Malkki, the author of this passage, expresses concern that the problem is laid at the door of bodies and minds of refugees rather than "in the political oppression or violence that produces massive territorial displacement of people" (Ibid.).

What makes it difficult for us to implicate the system that is the root cause of displacement and suffering? In this chapter, I engage with this question in relation to Sultan's life narrative.

Sultan is a 32-year-old single mother who claimed refugee status in Canada. Her life, not unlike those of other participants in the study, has been governed by multiple structural factors. Following the disruption of her education during the revolution, she married an Iranian man who was living in Germany. The marriage came to an end owing to, in Sultan's words, "isolation and racism." Sultan decided to come to Canada for her 6-year-old daughter. But things did not work out as she had planned. All that she wanted to do here was work but instead she spent all her time and energy dealing with an unresponsive and insensitive system.

This chapter is divided into two parts. In the first part, we will look briefly at notions of territories and boundaries—notions that will help us to understand why displaced people are considered an anomaly to be controlled and managed. In the second part, we will read Sultan's text to gain insights on two interrelated issues: how institutions insulate themselves from blame, and how people establish points of intervention in the system. A concluding section explores the potential of such interventions for social change.

Territories and Boundaries
ೞ

Territories and boundaries are units through which we come to imagine nation-states whose terms of reference are framed by Western discourses and practices. Territories evoke notions of rootedness and belonging. Boundaries are socially constructed and they determine the institutional practices of "who gets in" and "who must be excluded." But these are invariably partial acts. Boundaries are continuously subject to pressure from movements of people, ideas, capital and goods. Boundaries are thus characterized by social and symbolic meanings that do not lend themselves to absolute definitions. In this light, anthropologist Mary Douglas made the observation that those people who cannot be contained within the seemingly tightly drawn boundaries of nation-states are considered as "matter out of place." Douglas focuses on the all-too-familiar example of dirt. She notes that our need to be dirt-free and tidy is not functional but carries a symbolic load; the presence of dirt stands for societal disorder. "Reflection on dirt," she notes, "involves reflection on the relation of order to disorder, being to non-being, form to formlessness, life to death" (1966, 5).

Douglas's epistemological insights have laid the groundwork for understanding the power of a nation-state. This power derives not from its political state—powerful as this may be—but from its infrastructure underpinned by a discursive ideology of classification and categorization. Within this hegemonic topography, "a particular kind of regime of order and knowledge is instituted, one which is at once politico-economic, historical, cultural, aesthetic and cosmological"

(Malkki 1995, 4). In Foucault's words, the national order of things constitutes "a naturalizing physics of power that is at once micro-political and monumental in scale" (cf. Ibid., 6).

This state of affairs explains why those who are uprooted from the unit of a nation-state are considered to be polluting and threatening. As outsiders, uprooted people bring into relief the fact that what is presented as natural is indeed socially constructed. As refugees occupy a non-classificatory status, they are subjected to political and medical gaze. As Malkki (Ibid., 7–8) has expressed it:

> Refugees are seen to hemorrhage or weaken national boundaries and to pose a threat to national security, as is time and again asserted in the discourse on refugee policy. Here, symbolic and political danger cannot be kept entirely distinct. Refugees are constituted, in Douglas's sense (1966), as a dangerous category because they blur national (read: natural) boundaries and challenge time-honoured distinctions between nationals and foreigners.

A second reason why we are not able to establish a co-relation between the system and displacement has to do with double standards evident in the Canadian example. At one level we evoke humanitarian discourse for admitting refugees into the country. Canada is signatory to the United Nations Convention and Protocol concerning refugees. Yet, at another level, a different script is at work. We are biased towards admitting three classes of refugees: those who are skilled—the cream of the crop; those who come from Eastern Europe (read: white); and those who enhance the compassionate/saviour image of Canada (Creese 1992, Razack 1998). The gendered script that emerges says that unless a woman can make a case of being oppressed by her culture and country, asylum is not granted. In not being able to speak about the history of colonialism and racism, she is rendered into an object on which is inscribed the message of "imperialist as saviour" (Razack 1998, 89).

The Canadian refugee policy is geared towards achieving credibility on two fronts: domestic and international. In the first realm, it attempts to appease the fear of Canadians for admitting too many "polluting" and hard-to-assimilate people; in the second realm, the policy attempts to bring to the fore the image of Canada as a caring and generous nation. This kind of power play has not worked because Canadian refugee (and immigration) policy is bogged down in "a bureaucratic nightmare" of red tape (Foster 1998). I present Sultan's story and palpable reality as a point of intervention into the classification discourse on refugees and the contradictory Canadian refugee policy.

Sultan's Story: On-the-Ground Experiences of a "Refugee"

❧

In presenting the story of one woman, I make a case for the potential of narratives to inform larger issues on citizenship and nationhood, both which are of concern to displaced people. I will argue that this potential cannot be conceived as operating merely in the resistance mode; neither can it be seen at a unilinear level. Rather, the scenario at work involves multiple contexts evoked by the narrative text. I have paid attention to narrative devices of metaphor, images, choice of words as well as the mapping of events through which the narrator endeavours to give depth and meaning to her story and develop a "viewpoint of what is a whole life" (Becker 1997, 3; also refer to Frank 2000, Good 1994). Pertinent to my focus is this question: To what extent are possible contexts re-mapped in the narratives of people who are rendered "refugees"?

Sultan's story reveals two scenarios: how she was rendered a refugee, and her attempts to reverse this label and resume a citizen's life within the nation-state of Canada.

❧ Starting Points: Locating Herself in History

Sultan's birth in 1960s Tehran took place under the Pahlavi regime (1926–1979) that had embraced Western models of economic and social development (Farr 1999, Sullivan 1998). This particular move had far-reaching effects as it called for transformation of society at many levels: cultural, institutional, religious and familial. For our purposes, it is important to note that economic development entrenched within the political system of a nation-state is gendered. In *Remaking Women: Feminism and Modernity in the Middle East*, Abu-

Lughod (1998) has identified three issues. First is the way in which women have become "potent symbols of identity and visions of society and nation" (Ibid.). Second is the issue of women's intervention in nationalistic debates on their rights and status, and the third concern is the Western narrative on Muslim women with the veil as the prime symbol (also see Hoodfar 1997, Ahmed 1992). For Sultan this larger narrative on modernity is illustrated by her experiences of marriage and migration.

Sultan was born into a family of three brothers and one sister. Her mother was a homemaker and her father was a bank clerk. Like her older siblings, Sultan decided to go to university but could not continue with her education: "All of my brothers and sisters have got a university degree but me, because by the time I finished high school, the revolution started and all the universities were closed. So I decided to work in a bank."

When the university reopened after two years (1981), an ideological shift had taken place. In the new Islamic Republic of Iran, the education system was geared towards the production of good citizens (read: good Muslims). Women as pillars of society were expected to give priority to motherhood. In Afkhami's words: "[T]he suitability of other activities can be judged more or less according to the degree to which they interfere with or draw women away from their family responsibilities (1994, 409). This gendered script included other dimensions such as the annulment of the Family Protection Law. "An unreformed Islamic law was instated, including polygamy, child marriage, father or guardian's control of the first marriage ...." and free divorce for men, but not for women (Ibid., 410). Women could not become judges "and were dismissed or hounded from many government positions" (Ibid., 410). With the 1979 state-imposed injunction on *hejab,* the message given to women was that their place was in the home. But this had the reverse effect. Sultan explained: "Parents felt more comfortable letting their veiled daughters participate in public activities. This is because other people would not recognize them and they were safe. Under the Shah when women did not wear the veils, they were more restricted as they could not go out freely."Although there are shades of opinion on the subject of the veil, participants of the study expressed consensus that women should be able to exercise choice. In the absence of choice, women resort to other means—a point brought home in the narratives of other women. We learn that when women were denied the opportunity to become judges or occupy other high-level positions, they became independent entrepreneurs (Afkhami, 1994). When the Republic fired female judges, some women lawyers "continued to practise in the name of male family members, others worked as legal advisors to companies, and women *Majles* [parliament] deputies fought for them" (Ibid., 17). The overall effect has been the development of an indigenous movement where women are actively campaigning for their rights in the press, the parliament and among the *qadi* (Islamic clergy). Women's political mobilization that received short-term support during the revolution has been channelled into multiple spheres: domestic, economic, political and legal, including everyday acts of resistance. During my short visit to Iran (08/1999) I participated in a number of discussions led by women in their homes. When one woman asked another if she would stay home if her husband so wished, she replied: "It is not subject to negotiation."

The above scenario indicates that women's struggles for their citizenship rights have multiple reference points determined by particular moments in their life cycles. Initially Sultan decided to locate herself within the home sphere of marriage and motherhood. Following the disruption of her education, Sultan worked in the bank for a couple of years and then got married to an Iranian engineer stationed in Germany. After four years of marriage, Sultan left her husband, returned to Iran with her newborn daughter and filed for divorce. The reason was not marital problems as one would anticipate; it was racism and loneliness she experienced in Germany.

> When I went back to Iran from Germany, I asked for divorce after five years. First, I did not want to divorce. My husband was an engineer and he was very busy in his work and I always was lonely. My only hobby was television and sometimes shopping. In Germany, people feel more homesick but in Canada you don't have that feeling. People in Germany are more racist and they don't accept other ethnic groups in their community. They ignore you when you go to the stores or they turn their backs to you when

they see you and in their newspaper they write that foreigners have to leave the country. Even for the educated people like doctors who are practising there or businessmen who are doing business for fifty years, they still have this problem. But if a person is from Poland and his grandfather was a German (mother pregnant from a German solider during the war), he will be accepted by the community as they believe his roots are German. ... There is some racism here but it is not like Europe.

The above narrative shows that the stress of everyday racism took its toll on Sultan's marriage. Assuming a normalized sense of assumptions and cultural practices, the force of racism is both powerful and pervasive (Bannerji 1995). Here the experience of loneliness must not be considered as an individualized problem. For an immigrant woman, denial of basic entitlements such as opportunities for social interaction amount to a structural violation of her rights (Jiwani 2001). Sultan explained that initially she tried to make contact with the neighbours. For her this was only natural. "My lifetime experience is that neighbours are your friends—your first relatives." Her neighbours ignored her repeated invitations to tea. This practice of exclusion can be explained with reference to Germany's immigration policy, which considers immigrants as perpetual strangers and foreigners.

The difference of race was not the only issue. Sultan is a Muslim and it is important to look at the issue of being a Muslim in Europe. Modood (1997) offers useful insights, noting that the Muslims have emerged as the Other in the European nationalist discourse partly due to historical reasons and partly due to their visibility. The power of this discourse can be gleaned from the fact that anti-Muslim sentiments are present in places where the physical presence of Muslims is negligible, as is the case in Scandinavia. The idea of Muslims as the "archenemy"—the Other—is perpetuated in academic writings and the media. These works, as McGowan has shown, "serve as a backdrop for much of the cultural or religious prejudice that Muslims encounter in the West" (1999, 216).

The premise of German immigration policy is that immigrants are "guest workers" who are expected to leave the country eventually, regardless of the length of stay. As Melotti has expressed it, "They are allowed to live in the country for lengthy periods, even generations, but this fact, at least in principle, does not entail any change in their status. Indeed the acquisition of citizenship by immigrants is not envisaged at all: naturalization is very difficult to obtain and even immigrant's children born in Germany remain foreigners—foreigners in their own land ...." (1997, 81).

Sultan brings to light two issues. The first concerns her divorce, which she does not attribute to personal problems as would commonly be assumed to be the case. She does not even talk about her husband except to say that he was very busy. It was her non-acceptance as an Iranian/Muslim woman in Germany that led her to ask for divorce. Second, she wastes no time in offering insights from her personal situation so as to include the plight of other ethnic minorities. By using the term "you" ("They ignore you when you go to stores or they turn their backs on you when they see you"), she converts a personal experience into a collective one. Her sketch of "foreigners'" life in Germany verges on testimonio. This term captures the interface between the speaking subject and the "absent polyphony of other voices, other possible lives and experiences" (Beverley 1992, 96).

Following her divorce, Sultan decided to leave Iran at a time when migration loomed large on the horizon. The metaphor that captures this trend is that of "travel." Other then the physical movement of crossing boundaries, travel evokes interstitial cultural spaces and homelessness-as-home, to use Ong's (1995a, 352) terms. However, this is not the script understood by people who police the borders. Their gendered understanding of the situation is that Iranian women like other non-Western women are fleeing an oppressive situation and seeking full emancipation in the West. But this is not Sultan's take on the situation. She does not present herself as "running away" from Iran. She merely came to Canada under the rubric of a "travelling nation"—to map the travel of [Iran] as a nation and of [Iranianness as a notion]. These terms used by the cultural theorist Puar (1994) suggest constitution of a subject or subjects and multiplicity of locations to "disrupt linear accounts of diasporic subject formation which privilege singular and unidirectional movement from (a usually problematic notion of) "home" to "not home."

Sultan had learned from friends and relatives that the official immigration channel was not open to her as a woman. This is true. The Canadian refugee (immigration) policy is heavily biased towards male migrants who can make an economic contribution to Canadian society (Hyndman 1999; Thobani 1999). As a single mother, Sultan's chances were even more remote as she and her daughter would be conceived as dependents. Sultan thus exercised the only option that was available to her: she entered Canada as a visitor and claimed refugee status. Yet, she had no intention of remaining within the confines of this category. Throughout the interview she repeatedly stated that once she was in Canada, the only thing she wanted to do was work: "I knew that I would have a hard time in Canada. I had prepared myself for all the difficulties if only I could work."

Immigrants/Refugees Should Hit the Ground Running

ঔ

Canadian immigration policy is informed by the need to recruit skilled labour—individuals who are expected to "hit the ground running" (Foster 1998, 78). This premise remains unchanged despite numerous revisions to the policy ranging from a pre-1967 closed period, to a post-1967 open policy, to a post-1978 restrictive policy, followed by the 1990s "designer" policy. This governing principle also applies to refugees. Looking at her own individual situation, Sultan did not think that it was a big deal for her to settle down quickly with only a little bit of help: six months of English language training and "any job that is available so that I can be independent of the system." In putting forward what she regarded as a simple plan, Sultan wanted to move away from the label of a "refugee" and move closer to meeting the refugee-policy goal of settling down quickly. But this was not to be the case.

"All that I wanted to do when I came to Canada was to work." To her great disappointment, Sultan discovered that work was out of the question until her refugee claimant status was settled. In her efforts to stand on her own feet as soon as possible, she tried to learn English and register for a training programme, both of which would help her get a job. But she could not register for any of the programmes as the system could not accommodate the time clash between her daughter's school hours and her own. This is because immigrant women have low priority: they are not considered to be breadwinners (Agnew 1996). Women thus find themselves waiting in long queues. In Sultan's words:

> One of the problems for Iranian people like me is getting into the job market. For example, I wanted to work but because of my refugee status, I was not cleared. So I was not able to work or do volunteering work. I have applied to several daycare [centres] on the North Shore, but my applications have not been accepted as I am required to be an immigrant. Now my refugee status claim has been accepted but it is still not enough to get a job.

Sultan had to go through a long and arduous process to gain access to social services. No one brought the booklet "Settlement Services in Canada" to her attention. She did not know where to look or whom to ask. She related the difficulties she faced in getting an appointment with a service provider. It took her close to six months before she realized that training courses were indeed available. She wanted to get training for high-demand jobs such as bookkeeping and computers. To her dismay, she found that there was a long waiting list and "this is an issue and a barrier for people like me who want to move quickly."

Migration is a major life event involving loss as well as regeneration. The loss occurs because of separation from family, absence of a familiar milieu, and often downward economic mobility. Regeneration constitutes the building of a new life. This continuum is uneven owing to societal hurdles and barriers. This is because migrants are primarily desired for their labour (skilled and unskilled) and also capital. Conceptually and empirically, migrants are considered to be males; females who wish to settle down independently are anomalous figures, and the social apparatus that would facilitate the process of settlement has yet to include the concerns and aspirations of women. The host country's expectations are that the immigrants should settle down quickly and not be a burden on the system. The migrant also desires the same thing. However, there are differences in perceptions. Sultan observes:

Of course everyone has a special problem. It is different for me than the seniors. For me, with a child, I want to be active. I don't want to stay home and the government pay for me. This does not give me satisfaction. I like to be active and do something for the community. I am a person who started work at the age of eighteen. I want to be active in my life.

While Sultan highlights her own situation, she is aware of the needs of other Iranian immigrants. In *The Wounded Storyteller*, Frank echoes this sentiment: "Storytelling is for another just as much as it is for oneself. ... The moral genius of storytelling is that each, teller and listener, enters the space of the story for the other" (1995, 18). Sultan's understanding of waged work (telling her story) highlights this situation further. Sultan does not see work in a parochial sense of having a job. For her, work is a means to do something for the community, and to maintain integrity and dignity of self. It is also a means for maintaining continuity at the most fundamental level: "I have worked all my life and I want to continue to do so." While waiting to get into a training course, Sultan decides to learn English as a second language. She encountered another problem common to women striving to strike a balance between family and education/career. Her daughter attended school from 9 to 3 p.m. The English classes are held in the afternoons. If she attended the classes, she would not be able to pick up her daughter after school.

I spoke to my worker about this issue and I asked her to do something about this, but she did not agree to do anything. So these are the problems that I have and they do not allow me to move forward. My daughter is 7 years old and she is in grade one.

If the state's desired goal is to have the newcomers "hit the ground running," why is Sultan's wish to work not accommodated? Why is her reasonable request for daycare not taken into account in the light of the fact that the skills she would acquire would enable her to work? Why does she have to wait for a long time before she can take a training course? Are these not the measures that make it possible for newcomers to become independent of the social service system? Our response to these questions requires that we take a detour for a closer look at two gendered scripts: settlement services and the refugee hearing process.

Gendering Resettlement Services
❧

British Columbia Newcomers' Guide to Resources and Services (January 2000) states that immigrant settlement agencies are geared, among other things, to help new immigrants and refugees find jobs, locate appropriate housing and learn English. Under the headings health care, citizenship, banking, working, driving, child care, education, the legal system and so on, the *Guide* continues to reinforce the idea that help is available to newcomers and all they need to do is contact the appropriate agency. There is no mention made of the specific needs and aspirations of women except in the images of women scattered in the *Guide*. Under the section "The First Few Days," three African women are depicted walking with their children. Under the subheading "Climate," another picture shows a woman dressing her child for winter weather; under the subheading "Public Health," a white community health nurse is seen weighing a newcomer's baby. The picture of a woman using a computer is included in the section "Working." This is the extent to which gender issues receive attention.

To make gender more visible, it is necessary for us to explore such themes as "the material involvement of so-called Third World women in the world system, the interaction of gender politics with anti-colonial, post-colonial and liberation politics, and the relationship of gender to race, imperialism and cultural diversity" (De Groot 1996, 31). The following discussion is a modest contribution to this challenging task.

The first two pictures of "mother and child" reinforce the misplaced Western notion that a woman's place is in the home. In her seminal work, *The Renaissance of Women*, Smith (1984) observes that the Renaissance, referred to as the "extraordinary flowering of brilliancy," was essentially a male affair. Women were relegated to the private realm of family and domestic life. To make things worse, this realm was appropriated by the public and male market sphere that took over women's work in such areas as production and healing. Fox-Genovese (1991) has noted that despite women's mass presence in the labour force today, they are still primarily perceived to be "at home."

A different scenario prevails for immigrant and refugee women. These women form part of the global feminized workforce where their underpaid but vital work is barely noticed. Yet, discursively, non-Western women are perceived to be oppressed and confined to the domestic sphere. This is because non-Western women are subject to re-presentation while Western women engage in a game of self-presentation (Mohanty 2003). But this demarcation works against advancing the interests of all women. The imperialist gaze framing non-Western women as oppressed is cast to make white women believe that they are indeed liberated. The implications of the mother-at-home discourse demarcates women's lives in such a way that the domestic world is severed from the public world of waged work to the disadvantage of all women.

As female newcomers are largely sponsored, they come into the country with considerable disadvantage as they are not entitled to the service programmes geared for "male breadwinners." Their access to English language and job training programmes is often through the side door—special resource-strapped services. Second, is the shuttlecock game played by the three levels of government: federal, provincial and municipal. This scenario is voiced by service providers: "They [federal government] say that it is not their responsibility to fund this programme; sometimes they say that they can only fund a programme partially." The provider explained that they only get limited and partial support. In the case of the much-needed ESL programme for some of the post-revolution Iranian women, the bare-bones funding—a twelve-hours-a-week coordinator supported by a team of voluntary teachers—is not sufficient. Also, as daycare is not provided, some of women, like Sultan, are left with no alternatives. Third, massive restructuring and downsizing of social service programmes since the 1980s has had major impact on settlement services. The peripheral location of settlement services means that this sector is among the first to feel the financial axe. The impact on the already marginalized immigrant women is profound. They face greater isolation and are further pushed into the domestic sphere or compelled to take on low-paying no-fringe-benefits work, as was the case with the majority of the participants at the time of our study. The female newcomer's confinement within the home sphere or within labour ghettos is not exclusively a function of their lower status emanating from their own communities—a point of view advocated in the West. Their status is determined by institutional and societal barriers in their country of resettlement.

The above scenario explains why Sultan is not able to access either a training or an English language programme despite her strong desire to work. "I did not come to Canada to stay at home. I do not want to be on social assistance." Consider the strategies from the *Guide* that Sultan was encouraged to look at by her social worker.

In the section "Finding a Job" (2000, 52), a prospective worker is asked to check the computerized job listings at the Human Resources Development Centre (HRDC), to use newspapers and personal contacts to locate job openings, to apply to the personnel departments at various places, and to phone and visit companies among other things. The common ground and ideology that bring these strategies together is that of individualization. Feminist scholars across the globe have noted the multiple ways in which this ideology isolates women and undermines their potential to advance their interests. Commenting on the Middle-Eastern scenario, anthropologists Abu-Lughod (1998) and Friedl (1991) state that the loss of female-centred networks, brought about by capitalistic developments, have severely disadvantaged women. Consider the paths that Sultan explored in the way of getting "anything, any job that will get me out of the house—even volunteer work." HRDC was out of the question for her as it was far from her place of residence. And she had minimal personal contacts, as is evident from her observations:

> In Iran we had a very close family relationship. But in Canada, even if you have family but the relationship is not that close. In Iran the relationships are warmer and closer but not here. Maybe it is related to a weekly busy schedule that everyone has here and don't have time for each other. In Iran, family and friends put lots of time for each other, and try to solve their problems together. So those who come here, will be hurt emotionally a lot. When I came here, anytime

I needed something, I asked my two sisters to help me. But after a while, they told me that I have to take care of my work and they cannot be with me. First, I found it very hard but then I noticed that I am able to solve my problems although it was very hard. It is hard, when you do it by your own self and you are lonely.

At issue is the fact that the sociocentric relationships valued by newcomers have not made their way into the service system.

The *Guide*'s section on "Finding a Job" also includes the category Employment Programmes. It states: "There are courses to teach you how to look for a job. There are also job-training courses." Further on in the booklet, there is information on "English classes for adults": "There are many English classes available for adults to learn to speak, read, and write English" (Ibid., 77). The section then continues to explain that newcomers are eligible for free government-sponsored ESL classes, and furthermore that subsidy is available for low-income newcomers who may want to attend classes at a college or school. It then states that other community groups (including churches) may also provide classes. As we flip through the *Guide* we are informed about the availability of child-care services and subsidy for low-income families (Ibid., 69–72). All these sections were of great interest to Sultan: these are the facilities that would have enabled her to "move forward." But this was not the case. Sultan was not able to use any of these services. As noted above she was on waiting lists for ESL and job training programmes. When an ESL spot became available, she was unable to register owing to the fact that there was no one to take care of her daughter after school.

The absent-presence of women (their images are used for political gains: they must remain home or take up low-paid work) must be corrected but not in the sense of add-women-and-stir. As Hill Collins (1990/2000) has argued, women must be seen as producers of knowledge and theory that actively grapple with central questions of their lives. For this to happen, women must have an epistemological space, one that is "designed to challenge, extend and transform existing gender-blind, masculine scholarship" (De Groot 1996, 30). De Groot suggests three strategies: recuperation of women's knowledge and understanding of the world; valorization of women's work and activities; and transformation that would reverse gender-blindness. This framework would subvert the public versus private divide that has not advanced the interests of women in any part of the world (Fraser 1989).

In discussing the fundamental issue of a woman not being able to learn English or undertake a training programme because of structural constraints, Sultan establishes her own point of intervention. She tells her own story, which brings home the palpable reality of life that should register in a listening community. It does not take much imagination to enter Sultan's world, which is all too human: she is a newly arrived immigrant who has great desire to work and raise her daughter.

ຄວ Every Picture Tells a Story of Omissions and Suggests Possibilities for Change

I now draw upon a second example of health from the *Newcomers' Guide* (2000) to elucidate Sultan's embodied take on this subject. I reiterate the point that my focus on the *Guide* is governed by the fact that it reflects societal attitudes towards newcomers. The *Guide* per se is not the object of critique.

The first page in the section on health care depicts a picture of a white male doctor examining an elderly Sikh male. There is no woman present in this picture. The picture reveals and conceals. Our reading must therefore take into account multiple perspectives. For the immigrant settlement service workers, the picture is meant to give one message: namely, that health services are available to newcomers (including refugees). Medical anthropologists and Third World feminists suggest that we read a second Orientalist script (Scheper-Hughes 1992, Good 1994, Das et al 2001). According to this frame, the West positions and presents itself as superior—developed as opposed to the "underdeveloped Third World, the original home of the newcomers." Commenting on this scenario, Razack (1998) has cogently argued that Third World refugees are profiled as people fleeing from chaos and uncivilized conditions. Their migration to the West is then read in terms of them wanting the services unavailable in their home countries. Hence the phrase "immigrants and refugees are a drain on our system." What we do not want to (re)member (historical amnesia) is centuries of colonial and neocolonial exploitation that continues to drain the non-Western world of its resources (Farmer 2003, Kleinman et al. 1997).

A second reading of the picture highlights two more issues. The first relates to the dominance of biomedical technology, a symbol of which is the stethoscope controlled and solely used by the medical practitioner. Lock (1993), for example, notes that empiricist orientation of biomedicine leans towards fragmentation, measurement and abstraction of what otherwise is a palpable reality. This orientation invariably excludes and devalues the subjective experiences of the patients. The second issue is that the patient is a racialized person. As such his objectification is more acute. In her work on Cambodian refugees in California, anthropologist Aihwa Ong notes that the U.S.-bound refugees are subject to health-screening process that includes age-specific immunization as well as X-rays for tuberculosis. "Those with active or suspected active TB were placed in quarantine and not allowed to leave for the United States until deemed cleared" (1995b, 1245). This extensive screening process is put into place because of the socially constructed perception that "refugees are carriers of exotic and mysterious diseases" (Ibid., 1245). The script of pathology is also expressed in the *Guide*. It states: "Sometimes immigrants encounter emotional problems. They may feel homesick, afraid, forgetful, or hopeless" (2000, 36). In the light of these findings (also reported in other works), the picture of the white medical practitioner examining a Sikh newcomer cannot simply be read in terms of "availability of health services" for newcomers. As we shall note through Sultan's case, health services are *not* available and accessible to all newcomers.

My third reading of the picture is a gendered one. Joanna De Groot (1996) argues that gender should not merely be added to a particular field of study. Gendering of a particular field, she observes, can only take place if women's issues are included conceptually, methodologically and empirically. This approach suggests that if we were to add the image of a female newcomer into the picture, the gender bias in the *Newcomers' Guide* (this goes for the gender-blind literature too) would not disappear. Including a mere picture of a woman in the health section of the *Guide* will not suffice.

Let us now turn to Sultan's narrative for more insights.

I noticed that there is no equality in many aspects for people. For example, medical insurance. I have been asked to pay $64. I talked to my worker that I cannot afford this money and she suggested that I have to phone them. After I phoned medical care, they asked me to call the worker. So I don't know who is in charge for these type of things.

The difficulties that Sultan encounters in getting medical coverage are due to the fact that only government-sponsored refugees are eligible for Medical Service Plan (MSP). Refugee claimants may apply for an "interim federal health card" issued by Citizenship and Immigration Canada (*Newcomers' Guide* 2000, 32–33). This is a lengthy process and introduces another bureaucratic level, adding more pressure for a person already dealing with the difficult task of settling down, individually and without much community support.

Having made her case, Sultan critiques the system with a caveat that there is abuse of the system: "Unfortunately some of the people under the welfare abuse the system, for example they work illegally while having an indirect income." Note that her usage of the term "abuse" includes members of the public, and not just refugees. Sultan bemoans the fact that because of this abuse innocent people are targeted. Like Foster (1998), she suggests that the real source of abuse is not the people but the system itself. Bureaucratic systems invite abuse. Sultan then talks about inequality. She states that some people who had come to Canada as refugee claimants received MSP. "As I said, there is no same rule for everyone. A lot depends on who the worker is. Workers do what they want." She draws on a second example concerning legal aid. Her worker informed her that legal aid was not available anymore, but then Sultan found out that her friend had got one. "So there is no equality. This country is supposed to be a democratic country, but it is not."

We may note that Sultan does not look at equity issues in abstract and idealistic terms. It would be helpful to look at how equity is defined by the Canadian state. We must first recognize the fact that the Canadian government has been an active participant in several international declarations on human rights. Two major ones are the Universal Declaration of Human Rights and the International Convention on the Elimination of All Forms of Racial

Discrimination. Canada's ratification of these declarations would suggest that the country is committed to advancing an equitable society free of discrimination and racism.

Following the repatriation of the *Constitution Act* in 1982, Canada has enshrined the Charter of Rights and Freedoms (Henry et al. 1995, Agnew, 1996). The most significant equality provision is found in section 15 of the Charter under the "equality rights" clause. This clause prohibits discrimination based on "race, national or ethnic origin, colour (or) religion, among other factors, and ensures equal protection of the law" (Henry et al. 1995, 261). The recognition of societal inequalities is considered as an important first step. However, the Charter has been faulted for its vague definition of "discrimination," leaving this task to the court. Within the courts, the process of interpretation invariably takes an arduous course. Furthermore, the Charter has been deemed inadequate for addressing racism. This is because the Charter does not require governments to work towards racial equality. As Henry et al. have noted: "Thus, a government that did absolutely nothing about racial equality would be in full compliance with the Charter" (261). The very act of enshrining the equality-rights clause is based on the assumption that "equality exists; only lapses from it need to be addressed" (Ibid.). These observations point to the reality that those who are subject to discrimination have no established recourse. The Charter's outward commitment to equality exists in a vacuum as there is no infrastructure that could implement its principles. Noting the fact that legal recourse requires resources that minorities rarely have access to, Henry et al. make the apt comment that "... justice is economically inaccessible" (262).

The first scene that Sultan introduces concerns a sick child: her daughter. She explained that her temporary medical coverage had expired and her application for another one was caught in the bureaucratic maze. During this time her child came down with a high fever.

I have my medical care card now. But I am not sure if it is still valid. Otherwise, I don't know what I would do if my child became sick. The last time, I received a letter with the expiry date of March 30th and if I don't pay my insurance, it will be cancelled. I sent a letter that I cannot afford it. Now I am worried because I don't know if I am covered or not. One day it happened. I remember that my daughter was sick and she had fever. I was not covered. I phoned my worker and she told me to take her to the hospital downtown. I could not get there, it was very far and it was difficult to take her in the rain by bus to downtown. I went to North Shore Health and they did not accept her too. So I took her to an Iranian doctor on the North Shore.

The insurance does not pay for all the medication. It just pays for antibiotics [prescribed drugs]; so I have to pay for everything like anti-fever pill. Fortunately so far we have not been that much sick. You sometimes can make an appointment and discuss it with the worker and in case of approval then it will be paid. But it is not always possible as you are sick and you don't feel well enough to go there. Emotionally I am hurt. I am always asking God to keep us healthy and not become sick. I understand that there are people who are abusing the system and they have to be careful. But it is hard for those who are in real needs.

"Narrative is not simply that which is present in a completed story, whether a written text, a folk tale, or a story as told or performed. In order to constitute a narrative, the story must be appropriated by a reader or an audience," writes Byron Good (1994, 143). Good's work suggests a two-fold process: the what and the how of narrating. Sultan engages in both the processes simultaneously. While she tells her story, she draws in the reader. She accomplishes this task through depiction of a scenario that the reader can relate to: a sick child. Her act of relating the difficult task of travelling in a bus with a sick child on a rainy day implicates the system.

The mother-daughter story is bound to evoke some kind of response. But this universal image, as Malkki notes, has been used extensively to depict the situation of refugee women: "Having looked at photographs of refugees over several years, one becomes aware of the perennial resonance of the woman with her child" (1995, 11). Sultan steers clears of what Malkki refers to as "universalism of bare humanity" (12); the latter suggests a negative portrayal of women as people who have lost their culture and identity. Sultan in fact brings to light the political economy of displaced people, infusing it with human agency—an aspect that forms an integral part of her life narrative.

Sultan's testimonio is not only that of a displaced person depicting the absent polyphony of other voices with similar stories but also a critique of the larger system. She poses a challenge to service providers and policy makers. But this challenge cannot be read without "listening to and conversing with the myriad voices in civil society," as the subaltern writer Ranjit Guha expresses it. Admittedly, these voices are barely audible in the face of immensely powerful discourses of the state—discourses that are entrenched in the everyday practice of institutions. Guha (1996, 3) captures the task that lies before us:

> These are small voices which are drowned in the noise of stasis commands. That is why we don't hear them. That is why it is up to us to make that extra effort, develop the special skills and above all cultivate the disposition to hear these voices and interact with them. For they have many stories to tell.

If we were to pay close attention to what Sultan is saying, this is what we would hear: Why is it so difficult for someone like me to get a job in Canada? I am willing to go for training and learn the language. A job will allow me to become independent of the system. This is what you would like me to do. Why are there so many obstacles in achieving this basic goal? I have a child and all that I want to do is take care of her and work. I want to remain active— this is what all people desire. Why are you making it so difficult for me to have access to services that we are entitled to as refugee claimants? You have a system that is being abused and I understand that you have to be careful, but this does not mean that you should make life difficult for those of us who are in real need.

In narrating her experiences, Sultan continues to include others— refugee claimants, Iranian newcomers and people in general—conveying the message that her story is everyone's story. This is the point of view that Trinh T. Minh-ha, writer and filmmaker, subscribes to: "The story depends on every one of us to come into being. It needs us all, needs our remembering, understanding, and creating what we have heard together to keep on coming into being. The story of a people" (1989, 119).

In her account, Sultan moves back and forth among her personal experiences, those of other Iranian immigrants, and those of people as a whole. The term *testimonio* captures this orientation. By definition, this term refers to a narrative told in the first person "by a narrator who is also the real protagonist or witness of the events he or she recounts, and whose unit of narration is usually a 'life' or a significant life experience" (Beverley 1992, 92–93). Testimonio has a representational value and as such it differs from a conventional narrative. Other than affirming her life narrative, Sultan "evokes an absent polyphony of other voices, other possible lives and experiences" (96).

Before we move on to the next section, let us accomplish the task that we undertook earlier on, and that is to establish ways and means through which we can include "the picture" of a woman in the health section of the *Newcomers' Guide* (2000). So far we have established three points: first, that empirical visibility of women will serve no purpose. As anthropologist Henrietta Moore (1988) has noted, the main issue is not that of empirical inclusion but that of representation. Second, unless women are included at a structural level where conceptual, methodological and empirical issues converge, their gains will remain fragile; the third task before us is to reject universal images such as a "refugee woman with a child." Lucy Lippard's (1992) work on photographs is of value as it brings to light new perspectives.

Lippard suggests that we should learn to read the space between the moment when a picture is taken and the moment in which we view it now, from our present location. A double and even a triple take is a good starting point. In the case of the health picture in the *Guide*, the first take involves making mental notes of words and images evoked by the picture: a turbanned Sikh, a white male doctor, a stethoscope, and also the omission/erasure of a female figure. There is no eye contact (interaction) between the two human figures. The caption captures our attention. It states: "B.C. health insurance, Emergencies, Doctors, Prescription Drugs, Dentists, Public Health Units." The message is to the effect that these services are available

to newcomers and that is why they are included in the *Newcomers'*
Guide.

The second take on the picture derives from Sultan's experiences;
as we listen to her story, we begin to realize that the picture has
cracks. The third take begins when we actually enter into her space.
It is a moment of *intersubjective encounter*, which, according to Lippard,
"commemorates a reciprocal moment ... where the emphasis is on
interaction and communication; a moment in which subject and
object are caught in exchange within shared time, rather than shouting
across history from their respective peaks" (37). While Lippard
cautions us that this may be an ephemeral moment, it allows us the
opportunity of "seeing for ourselves, the way we never would see
for ourselves, which is what communication is about" (43).

We have so far established two interrelated modes through which
the possibility of a mutual encounter between the narrator and the
researcher/reader can be considered. The first is reading the narrative
(the reader's response) through generous contextualizing, and the
second is viewing a picture or photograph through multiple takes.
For further exploration of the transformative potential of these
modes, we will read and "picture" Sultan's account of the refugee
hearing process.

The Refugee Hearing Process
౮౦

As I said I am living in Vancouver for two years. It took me more
than a year to go through the process of my court, and it was a
very difficult period of my life. Unfortunately, as many refugees
are coming to this country and it make lots of stress on the
government. You have to go through that difficult process of the
court. I feel much better emotionally as my refugee status is
approved. I am more established now.

Since I applied for refugee status, I have had hearings four times.
Every time I prepared myself to answer the questions for the court,
it cancelled due to absentee of the judge or not having the empty
room, and then I had to go back after two months. You can imagine

how my mind was filled with worries until the next court hearing. In my court, they questioned me for eight hours and because still they were not satisfied and my situation was not clear for them, then they kept it on hold. They were curious to know about my personal life but anyway it was solved and I was accepted as a refugee here. I was dreaming the court, and all the questions that they raised, for two to three weeks. After the approval, I started to work on my other things such as welfare, English class, Medical Care, etc.; but unfortunately everything takes so long here. They are not as fast as they are supposed to be. For example, I wanted to see my worker and she gave me appointment twenty days later.

Life would be much easier for me if I could find a job. I would like to be active in my life and have a job.

Time looms large in the above narrative. Out of the two years that Sultan has been in Vancouver, one year was taken up by the refugee hearing process. Sultan's views of this occurrence may be understood at three levels. First, she is keenly aware of the abuse of the refugee system; in this regard, she positions herself to participate in the debate on this topical issue. As I write, the *Globe and Mail* (Dec. 11, 2000) has published an article titled "Refugee claimants inundate Ontario." The subject of the article, written by Andrew Mitrovica, concerns claimants flooding into Canada from the United States. The article lists the source countries of the twenty-five to thirty claimants: Argentina [main source country], Sri Lanka, Colombia, Pakistan and Turkey; it predicts that by the end of the fiscal year, April 2001, the total number would be 10,000 compared with 1,536 in 1998–99. While the media have created the floodgate argument (the Third World knocking on the doors of the First World), the picture is more nuanced. In this particular case, the rise in the number of refugees is attributed to the fact that the United States has implemented a visa-waiver pilot programme for Argentina and other designated countries. Another reason cited for the rise was rumours about proposed changes that would make Canada's immigration policy more stringent, purportedly to crack down on immigrants and refugees with criminal records. As far as Canada is concerned, its refugee policy has been a source of friction between two polarized groups: those who believe that the existing system must be tightened to prevent the entry of terrorists and war criminals, and others who subscribe to the idea that the majority of the refugee claimants are hardworking people who make an enduring contribution to the Canadian society.

Sultan presents herself as a participant and not an object of this debate. She states that the government is subject to stress in having to deal with a large number of claimants. She is also aware that the system may sometimes be abused, which results in a more vigorous hearing process being put in place to eliminate bogus claims. But at the same time, she expresses her experiential understanding of what it is like for a claimant to go through a system whose primary focus is a suspicion that the claimant is not genuine in her intentions to become a law-abiding citizen. The system is also resource-deprived— a reflection of the ambiguities surrounding the status of refugees, as discussed at the beginning of this chapter.

On the one hand, refugees help to boost the humanitarian image of Canada; on the other hand they are perceived as a burden. We may also note that in the screening process, the economic criteria are factored in and priority is given to those refugees with professional qualifications. Discursively, refugees are people who are considered as "matter out of place" and therefore a threat to national boundaries that have always been fragile; nation-states are built on the principle of exclusion of minorities, including women (Yuval-Davis, 1997).

In order to illustrate her plight as a person dealing with an insensitive system (for reasons mentioned above), Sultan decides to frame her narrative in terms of time. Time, despite the fact that it is socially constructed and culturally experienced, constitutes an arena that all human beings can relate to at a personal level; it is an embodied experience. We all know what it is like to wait for an outcome that for some people may be a life and death issue. It is at this level of engaging the reader that Sultan relates her experiences: her hearing was scheduled four times and cancelled because of the non-availability of the judge or a room. She had to wait for two months. Then, when her hearing did take place, she was questioned for eight hours. Even then a decision was not reached until more information was gathered on her personal life. This process had an emotional impact on Sultan: "I was dreaming of the court. I could not concentrate on anything else. I was emotionally drained." Her experience of waiting did not come to an end at the point when she was granted the refugee status. She had to go through a second round of waiting when applying for various benefits to which she was entitled. At the time of writing (ethnographic present), she is still waiting to get into an ESL class.

In the above section, I have interpreted Sultan's account as she related it and the way I have understood it. I have also found it necessary to include the larger contexts to make the connection between her narrative and the political economy of resettlement. Our next step is to engage in a second reading of this account and pay special attention to the scripts that are not related but nevertheless present.

Which Scripts Are Told and Which Scripts Are Silenced?
౭౦

Ranjit Guha suggests that we should learn to distinguish between a dominant version of events and the small voices of history. The authority of the dominant version is built into the structure itself; it has a certain order of coherence and linearity. This order dictates the inclusion of some elements and the exclusion of others. The process is determined by the targeted outcome. For Guha, the impact of the small voices can only be felt if it can force the dominant version to "stutter in its articulation instead of delivering an even flow of words ...." (1996, 12). Let us then examine the interplay between the dominant script and its subaltern and gendered variation.

A cursory glance at the global scenario reveals people on the move for a myriad of reasons. But the mobility of people is policed at the national borders because there are only some people who are welcome, namely, those who are "perceived" to be contributing members of the host (Western) society, those who can fill empty slots in the labour force ghettos. What happens to people who find themselves excluded because they do not meet the host country's admission criteria? What happens in a situation of political upheavals, persecution and economic debacles? Increasing visibility of these displaced persons has prompted United Nations to adopt guidelines for refugees. According to the United Nations Convention and Protocol, a refugee is defined as a person who is seeking asylum from persecution based on race, religion, nationality and membership in a particular social group. These broad categories do not include gender. Canada has adopted the UN Convention and Protocol, and to reverse the gender imbalance it has introduced a series of Guidelines for the Immigration and Refugee Board (IRB).

The Guidelines are based on the fact that women are unable to seek asylum for gender-based persecution under the existing UN criteria. The Guidelines enable women to make their case if they are subject to familial or state-based acts of violence; they go so far as to include *fear of persecution* (Razack 1998, 103).

The Guidelines constitute an important step for women as they acknowledge the reality of gender-based persecution. The fact that this document is specially prepared for the adjudication process of the Immigration and Refugee Board means that elements of the Guidelines can be put into practice. While we are cognizant of the goodwill invested in the formulation of the Guidelines, however, its implementation is problematic.

There is marked absence of the "small voice" in the implementation phase of the Guidelines. Let us for a moment look at some examples suggested by Razack (1998). This author observes that a review of the IRB female refugee hearing process revealed that the officials were not always respectful of the claimants and operated with skeleton information about the claimants' countries of origin. To rectify this situation, educational sessions were recommended for members of the panel, with emphasis on culture. But critical scholarship suggests that this is not a cultural or gender-sensitive issue. What is required is a vigorous and analytical understanding of the country's socioeconomic conditions (Razack 1998, Ong 1995b).

Inclusion of the socioeconomic script of the claimants' countries of origin would mean laying bare the colonial and neocolonial legacies that have contributed to gender persecution in the first place. This point has a bearing on Sultan's life. The West is implicated in the 1978–79 Iranian Revolution; in its intent, the Revolution was an attempt to reverse the foreign control of over a century of the

Iranian economy, first by Britain and later by United States (Farr 1999). Sultan poignantly expressed this point: "Were it not for Queen Elizabeth and President Clinton, I would still be in Iran." Likewise Razack observes that the West's exploitative activities have contributed to the production of the world's refugees—a point that was brought home to us in the displacement of over one million Afghani people in the wake of the post–September 11, 2001 U.S.-led attack on Afghanistan.

There does not exist a space where the script of the small voice—the colonial narrative of exploitation (material and epistemic)—can be articulated. The refugee hearing process, then, can only take place within the narrative of cultural Othering where "we see ourselves as saving her [the claimant] from a dysfunctional overly patriarchal state" (Ibid., 04). Herein lies the paradox. In their attempt to include gender, the Guidelines contribute to sustaining the gendered colonial subtext of women fleeing from patriarchal violence believed to be embedded in their cultures and communities.

There are two more points related to gender inclusion in the Guidelines. First, the inclusion is marginal and nonstructural, as the UN Convention and Protocol does not recognize gender as a separate category. This form of structural exclusion translates into fragile gains as the Guidelines can be subject to changes that may not favour women. Second, women's multiple roles as sisters, wives, mothers, workers and citizens are subsumed under the dominant paradigm of gender persecution. The message conveyed here is that all women are subject to violence; to add insult to the injury, women's culture and traditions are identified as the source of this violence, overlooking the exploitative workings of the neocolonial and global economy noted above.

We do not know the content of Sultan's argument in the court. She decided not to talk about the basis on which she was granted refugee status. As Visweswaran has informed us, women's silence is a marker of agency and we cannot assume the willingness of women to talk. But what we can do is pay attention to why and when women talk (1994, 52), to which I would add the what and the how of women's speech.

In the above section, we have attempted to "read" Sultan's story, paying close attention to the content that she has highlighted and the form she has given to it. Our reading of her story is guided by a broader framework of dominant discourses and small voices. Our final task is to see if we can "picture" the court scene (refugee hearing) in order to create a space where we can begin to explore the issue of accountability, thereby inserting ourselves into the picture to examine our own complicity in sustaining power imbalances.

Lippard suggests that when we look at pictures and photographs, we must learn to crack their surfaces and break them open "to get at the living content that has been erased from our history books" (1992, 15). If we were given the opportunity to photograph the court scene, the profile that would come to light would be that of a woman facing members of the board. They have the privilege of asking questions, including personal and intimate details, for any length of time they choose (eight hours in Sultan's case). The claimant can only respond to the questions. Sultan is not given the space to ask questions or tell her story in her own terms. The political and social hierarchies that surround the refugee hearing process cannot be more pronounced. But we cannot close on this note. We must grasp the living content from Sultan's narrative to explore this question: To what extent is her story our story?

To think through this question, I am helped by sociologist Dorothy Smith's concept of texts. To begin with, a text is not an artifice but a product of local historicity. It is made in an actual setting by one or more people as part of a course of action. Furthermore, a text is read in time and in place and therefore it has the potential to enter into someone's course of action. A text can therefore have a speaking part. Smith's second observation concerns the use of language. In the Bakhtinian tradition, she notes that language is a shared enterprise. We use words to communicate and elicit a response from the listener/reader. One is thus positioned to take the word and make it one's own. As language has its source in real-life situations— the living content that we are seeking to identify in the picture—Bakhtin's words ring true: "Each word tastes of the content and contexts in which it has lived its socially charged life" (cf. Smith 1999, 148). Therefore, concludes Smith, our reading must enable us to escape from "the stasis of the text into the lived actuality" (Ibid.).

If we agree that to speak and to write are essentially dialogical acts to the extent that dialogue is worked into every word and sentence, the same principle applies to a photograph. There are no words or sentences but layers of meaning that can be arrived at if we remember that the person in the picture has a story to tell. The story must be told and the listening must take place, as Trinh Minh-ha (1989) reminds us; the question is, what do we do once we have listened? A socially and politically engaged response would be one viable step.

What we need to recognize is that Sultan came to Canada as a "refugee," as assuming this status was the only avenue open for her. But she did not want to be rendered a refugee per se. Her goal was to become independent through work, broadly defined to include elements of dignity and meaning. But her structural location in Canadian society, as an immigrant Muslim woman, rendered her powerless with minimal or no resources to attend to such building blocks as learning English and upgrading her qualifications. As a categorized refugee, Sultan is locked into a dependent position—essentially a maze of social services. The paradox of her being drawn into a system that has no resources to offer ("Be a guest in the house but there is no bed or food for you") may be explicated with reference to the insensitive policy orientations. The act of omission in the way of no or minimal social programmes for immigrant women are the result of policy decisions bolstered by the discourse of the Other; the Other in this case being a person or a group of people who have not been accorded civil, political and social rights that they are entitled to as citizens of a nation-state. In Canada, this discriminatory and racist practice is masked by discourses on multiculturalism and cultural diversity. The latter "helps to obscure deeper/structural relations of power, such as racism and sexism or racist heterosexism, both among women and the working class, and reduces the problem of social justice into questions of curry and turban" (Bannerji 2000, 38).

Economic and social justice issues suggested in the above observations are implicated in Sultan being rendered a "refugee." I have argued that the "refugee" status is not acquired at the time when a person leaves one's country but that is a function of the treatment accorded to these individuals upon arrival in the host country. (The term "host" is a misnomer as the host country [the West/global capitalism] is implicated in the displacement of millions of people [Malkki 1995]). Sultan assumed the legal status of refugee claimant to claim her rights (travel and travelling nation) to live in the West. Logically, this legal status should open into a community space of work and citizenship. But instead Sultan finds herself more confined; she ends up in the social service sector where she is rendered into a dependent status.

Through the act of storytelling Sultan engages with the system in a way that allows her to assume the role of a critic. This state of affairs comes about because struggle and suffering lead to the creation of voice and narrative power. As Frank has expressed it, the wounded need to become storytellers so as to recover their voices. Non-conventional channels may be deployed to engage the listeners. The silent language of the body has been identified as salient (Scheper-Hughes 1992, Frank 1995, Becker 1997): "... in the silences between words, the tissues speak" (Frank 1995, xii). Creative use of metaphors (Becker 1997), evoking reader's response (Good 1994, Frank 1995), working towards collaborative partnership (G. Frank 2000, Ong 1995a) and bringing to the fore broader contexts (Personal Narratives Group 1989) are other popular strategies that disadvantaged people use to come to voice and come to power through reconfiguration of dominant discourses. We have focused in this chapter on generous contextualization suggested by Sultan's framing of her story. The narrative contexts of life in Iran, departure, resettlement experiences (social services, refugee hearing process) have helped us to see that far from being the Other, refugees are people who seek basic entitlements accorded to other citizens. Rather than focusing on the bodies and minds of refugees, we need to pay closer attention to the system that displaces people in the first place— a point of view suggested in Sultan's narrative.

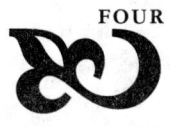

FOUR

Looking for Work:
Nadia's Story

Nadia and I met at the North Shore health advisory committee meeting. I had joined this group in the early years of my field research to get a sense of how immigrant and multicultural health issues were framed institutionally.[1] Nadia had joined the committee with the hope of finding work in her professional area of oncology.[2] Having been in Canada for six years, Nadia was desperate to get anything remotely connected to her area of expertise. During my subsequent meetings with her, I learned that other than her vigorous search for work, she was seeking answers to one particular question: Why is it so difficult for an English-speaking Iranian professional to work in Canada? She noted that the Canadian embassy had told her and her husband (an engineer) that "there would be no problems for them getting work in Canada." In this chapter, I give a long answer to Nadia's question. I show that the response cannot be framed in a linear mode; it must necessarily emerge from the genre of storytelling with its multifaceted potential for capturing the voices of research participants at many levels. Nadia had her own reason for sharing her story with the reader: she wanted people to recognize and validate her suffering, which was caused by her not being able to work in her area of expertise. For Nadia the issue was no less than her basic right to work and live with dignity.

As I began to think through Nadia's story, related to me over a period of fourteen months, the analytical paradigm of "intersectionality" came to the fore. This emerging paradigm suggests that "race," gender and class are intricately connected to the extent that a focus on one at the exclusion of others yields a distorted picture

(Bannerji 1995). But this is not the whole story and never can be if we want to pay close attention to the lived reality of people. The race/gender/class paradigm is limiting as it is grounded in the divisive Cartesian epistemology that invariably focuses on one category to the exclusion of others. Literature on race and ethnicity does not as a matter of course include gender issues, and likewise a focus on gender may exclude other categories. Furthermore this paradigm leans heavily on victimization with little room for consideration of human agency. My intent is not to undervalue the power of this paradigm, as it has effectively unmasked oppressive systems of power. However, I take one more step to ensure that the lived and storied reality of women and the "small voices" of civil society are not dismissed, because they have the potential to effect change. Both the scenarios—intersectionality and small voices—throw light on the question posed by Nadia as to why she is not able to find work in Canada. The small voices paradigm will help us (the readers) to understand who Nadia is in terms of historical and social trajectories. At this level we can appreciate Nadia's stature as a person and not merely as a socially constructed immigrant woman destined for a ghettoized labour force.

In my analysis, I remained close to the format of Nadia's story and divided the chapter accordingly. The first part deals with Nadia's account of erasure of her professional qualifications following her immigration to Canada—an aspect explicated through the paradigm of intersectionality. The second part profiles her lived reality in Iran—the small voices that Nadia herself presents to highlight her historical trajectory in terms of her sense of who she is as a woman. The conclusion explores the implications of the intricate relationship between the two paradigms.

The Intersectionality Paradigm: "Why Can I Not Work in Canada?"
ೞ

A cogent analysis of immigrant women and waged labour in Canada comes from the work of Roxana Ng. In her 1988 (2nd ed. 1996) study, Ng argues that the state plays a key role in placing immigrant women on the lower rungs of the labour force hierarchy. The state accomplishes this through two means: it establishes a gendered and racialized hierarchical structure, and it works through community agencies that it funds. Acting as agents of the state, the agencies then channel immigrant women into low-paid work.

Writing in the late 1990s, Joanne Lee comments on more recent developments. Like Ng, Lee examines the workings of community and social agencies operating under the changed climate of fiscal restraints. Faced with the demands made by the global market economy for debt reduction and mitigation of corporate taxes, the government has downsized the social service sector. As is invariably the case, those at the margins are affected the most, and such has been the case with female immigrants working in the "not-for-profit, community-based, multi-ethnic, and ethno-specific organizations and groups, as well as branches and divisions of mainstream institutions such as schools and hospitals" (1999, 97). Lee shows that the state uses gender and race categories to simultaneously marginalize the settlement sector and within it the immigrant female settlement workers. Within this under-funded sector, immigrant women's opportunities for career advancement are eroded. Moreover, the funding crunch creates a situation where the boundary between volunteer and paid work remains porous. Immigrant female worker's unpaid work is justified along the lines of this well-known script: immigrant women need to do voluntary work to gain Canadian experience. The institutionalization of volunteerism is paradoxical: "While these strategies offer opportunities to immigrant and refugee women to use their skills in the community, they also limit and channel these skills" (100). Their ghettoized status, as shown in Nadia's narrative, is sustained by racialized (it is all right for women of colour to work for nothing) and feminized (women are inclined by nature to undertake social service work) discourses.

What I have presented above are not merely case examples but representations of a growing body of work on the power and knowledge nexus of the intersectionality paradigm (Bannerji 1995, Jiwani 2001, Thobani 1999, Razack 1998, Dua and Robertson 1999, and Aylward 1999 among others). The focus here is to explain the structural locations of immigrant women in relation to a set of social relations and practices that have led to their marginalization. This body of work, I argue, must be examined in relation to the lived reality of women.

Forming part of the political economy of migration and of late global capitalism, the intersectionality paradigm has dominated the field to the extent that immigrant women's agency in negotiating their life situations in their adopted countries has received less systematic and theoretical attention except in the form of resistance strategies. For example, Bannerji's (1995) fine-grained analysis of sexual harassment of a Black Canadian woman does not include the issue of voice. The readers are not introduced to this woman's own understanding of the situation. What are her particular insights on social change? What kind of embodied knowledge does she have on the racist-sexist organization of the economy and its workplace?

My second example comes from Stevenson's (1999) work on First Nations Women.[3] This author argues that the collaborative hegemony of the church and the state have undermined these women's status and autonomy. It is only towards the end (the last two paragraphs) that we learn that First Nations communities did indeed resist total subjugation through healing and spirituality. How were the latter sustained? What analytical frameworks could explain the working of civil and small voices? (They are "small" because they are not heard.) The tension between the paradigm of intersectionality and that of civil voices requires more sustained attention if we are to avoid polarizing the lives of immigrant and aboriginal women as either victims of the system or individuals in control of their lives. To bridge the gap between the two paradigms, I explore the mediating role of storytelling. I show that the stories of marginalized people include both elements: structure and human agency, portrayed within nuanced contexts.

Nadia's story occupies a critical juncture: it is the story of a displaced life that is also gendered.[4] This means looking at epitomizing moments of who she is and what her life has been like prior to and upon migration to Canada. Iranian poet and writer Faraneh Milani exemplifies the complex lives of displaced women:

> I was immersed in discontinuities; engulfed in geographical, cultural and temporal exile. Neither the daughter of my mother nor the mother of my daughter, I felt suspended between the twentieth century AD and fourteenth-century Hegira. The gap between my mother and my daughter, products of different cultural experiences,

values, systems of signs, dreams and nightmares, had caused a
disturbing disruption in the matrilineal chain of my identity. I lived
surrounded by a past that was breaking up around me with violent
rapidity. (1992, xi–xii)

Nadia's narrative on who she is, how she came to Canada, her search
for work and how she fared as a daughter to a mother living in Iran
and a mother to a daughter (and a son) living in Canada highlights
the issues set out by Milani. Nadia's sense of identity—who she is/
was/could be—is tied to her desire to work in her area of expertise
as an oncologist.[5] I begin with a defining moment, when she crosses
the border into a new land.

Border Crossing

ೞ

On August 11, 1992, Nadia, accompanied by her husband and their
two children—a girl and a boy aged 17 and 15 respectively—landed
at Vancouver International Airport. Upon her arrival, she
encountered two lanes: Domestic and International. Since this was
her first trip to Canada, Nadia went into the international lane further
demarcated into two sections: Residents and Visitors. Nadia followed
the visitor's lane clutching her landed status papers. Residents with
Canadian passports are asked standard questions by the uniformed
immigration officials: "How long have you been out of the country?"
"Which places did you visit?" "What did you purchase?" These
seemingly benign questions carry the weight of legislation in terms
of who can (re)enter the country and under what conditions. As
Kumar has observed, the immigration officer takes the passport and
papers as a book: "Under the fluorescent light, he reads the entries
made in an unfamiliar hand under the categories that are all too
familiar. He examines the seals, the stamps, and the signatures on
them" (2000, 3). A ritual is set in place: the immigration officer asks
questions and listens to the responses, paying attention to the clothes
and the accent. If the responses match the officer's reading of the
passport and papers, the turnstile works in favour of the immigrants.

Interrogation to which new immigrants are subject forms part of the constitution of "hegemonic moments" where migrants are defined not as people coming from another part of the world but in relation to powerful frames of race, gender and class. These socially constructed categories give rise to the phenomenon of policed borders—borders so powerful that they may and often do assume symbolic and social forms when the person in question is from the non-Western world (Razack 1998).

Due to Nadia's class status of being a professional, like her husband, the interrogation that she was subjected to as a Muslim/Iranian woman did not begin at the time of her entry to Canada, but soon after. More important, it did not take place on a face-to-face level but indirectly through societal systems.

First Moments
ಐ

We came to Vancouver because a friend had informed us that this was a good place. We stayed for a few days in a motel and then rented an apartment at Mountview [an apartment complex where several Iranian families live]. My first crisis was to learn that my husband would not be able to work in Vancouver. For an engineer it is not easy to work in the city. He had to go to a small town. I stayed with the children. I did not want my children to live around other Iranian families. We moved to another part .... Once I settled the children in school, I started looking for work. But I was not successful. I was told I did not have the Canadian experience. I do not think anyone ever bothered to read my resume.

For the first three months, Nadia phoned every place where she thought she had a chance for a job. After that, she joined a three-week long job-finding class and

... that gave me information about resources and contact persons. I prepared my resume and a covering letter and I applied to many places for a job but no success. I got a volunteer research job at one place and then one day an advertisement in the *North Shore*

News about a computer course caught my eye. I applied for that
and I went through interviews and I was accepted. Before I got
this chance, I had to change my resume and "hide" my qualifications.
It was a nine-month full-time course. I learnt different computer
programmes and through that I was able to find a part-time job in
a seniors' organization. In that office, I worked hard. I experienced
discrimination and racism a lot. Emotionally, it affected me so
much so that last December it gave me almost a nervous
breakdown and I quit that job. I was able to get another part-time
job in a larger centre right away and I worked there for a year. I
really enjoyed working there. But it was not a full-time job. The
staff were really nice people, very supportive and I had great time
there. I still have close relationship with staff who recommended
me to a recreation centre for women.

As discussed above, Ng (1988/1996) documents the process
through which a community employment agency, through its daily
work, produces immigrant women as a labour market category. She
highlights a paradox: the agency that was established to advance the
interests of immigrant women in fact advances the state's agenda of
producing immigrant women as a labour market "commodity." Nadia
did not resort to an employment agency but she was not spared the
ghettoization of racialized women. Gender- and race-specific training
programmes were already in place and they carried out the work of
the agency along the lines suggested by Ng. Let us look more closely
at this aspect.

The training programme subtly channelled Nadia into the
marginalized service sector targeted for immigrant women—a
development that took place at the cost of erasing Nadia's
professional qualifications ("I had to change my resume to 'hide' my
qualifications.") The very fact that she could not get into a training
programme in her area of expertise illustrates the way in which Nadia
was channelled into low-paid work. Second, Nadia was slotted into
the niche created in response to the tight fiscal economic climate of
the 1990s: part-time no-benefits work in a marginal cash-strapped
service organization. Consider the following scenario.

Since the 1980s, the Canadian state has been part of the global
Structural Adjustment Program that has led to severe budget cuts in

the social service sector. The effects of this restructuring on the already-marginalized immigrant social service sector are pronounced. As Agnew (1996) and Lee (1999) have argued, the budget cuts not only have limited the capacity of service providers to offer much-needed programmes to those who need them the most, but have had a negative impact on the working conditions of the largely female immigrant settlement and social service workers. The latter are compelled to engage in overtime volunteer work without which the existing but fragile programmes could come to an end, resulting in the loss of even the existing low-paid jobs. Also, immigrant women hang on to whatever they have (part-time and volunteer work) with the hope that they will eventually find better paying and more stable work. This is the promise implied by the much-used and abused expression "You do not have Canadian experience." However, the prospect of finding better employment is negligible, as racialized women are systemically positioned to move within a lateral space with limited opportunities for advancement.

Although Nadia found that the staff treated her well in her second job, structurally it was was no different from her first job, in that it was low-paid ghettoized work. The subtext here is that there are a sizable number of Iranian consumers and volunteers involved in the programme because Iranians form the largest ethnic and religious minority on the North Shore. Nadia's work in the social service sector then was timely from the point of view of service organizations: she would and did attract more Iranian consumers as well as Iranian volunteers. As most of them were not fluent in English, Nadia offered the added asset of being bilingual. However, she was not paid extra wages for the two-way translation that she did for both the parties: the English-speaking coordinator of the programme and the Farsi-speaking consumers and volunteers. Nadia was in fact "used" on some occasions. She related that it put her in an awkward position. When it came to subsidizing low-income individuals, the programme's coordinator turned to her to determine if the Iranian applicants were genuine.

Nadia's placement in the social service sector did not even come close to the deficiency and dysfunctional discourse applied to many immigrant women: they do not speak English, they do not have the

Canadian experience, they are docile, and their qualifications are not up to Canadian standards. Nadia is a highly qualified medical professional who studied at a good university in Iran and is fluent in English. Before joining the service sector, Nadia had applied for further studies in her field of expertise at a university in British Columbia, but her application was not considered owing to "medical training strictures." Thus Nadia's interrogation—"Who is she?" with its implicit message of "Why has she come to Canada?"—began at the workplace and not at the time of border crossing. Within the framework of the intersectionality paradigm, this would be Nadia's whole story: a professional immigrant woman is subtly channelled into the ghettoized slot. Her waged or voluntary work fits well into the Canadian immigration policy geared to meet the labour market and voluntary-based needs of Canadian society. In the present-day fiscal climate of restraint, the labour market absorbs the low-paid work of immigrant women, which translates into work on three fronts: the labour force, the volunteer force and the domestic sphere.

In the process of looking for work and later working part time, Nadia cared for her two children in a new country where she fell into the category of "a single-headed household," although she is married. Other than mentioning the difficulties of becoming a virtual "single parent" because of circumstances, in her narrative Nadia does not dwell on this part of her life. Her primary focus was captured in the recurring statements variously expressed: "I worked hard for my career." "I am a professional woman." "My lifetime work has been taken away from me."

At the particular juncture of what is commonly referred to as "the downward mobility of immigrant women," Nadia talks about her life back at home. Her decision to share this part of her life with the reader shows that she did not accept the system's narrow definition of work (read: wages); neither did she accept the social construct of "an Iranian immigrant woman" (read: oppressed and passive). The civil-voice script that Nadia highlights is this: "I am more than a socially constructed immigrant woman." I present Nadia's narration of events in the form of the canvas of life, an apt metaphor for appreciating a lived life with its complexities and contradictions.

Section One: The Canvas of Life

Experiences of disruption are common among individuals attempting to create a new life. Gay Becker's work *Disrupted Lives: How People Create Meaning in a Chaotic World* exemplifies this narrative moment. Citing the case of Mrs. Zabor—an 82-year-old Hungarian refugee— this author notes how through skillful use of painting, this woman recreates "... her personal history, the canvas of her life. Small and fragile looking, her expressive hands move in the air as she moves from one picture to the next, in a continuous process of life reconstruction ...." (1997, 2).

Becker observes that the scenes from Mrs. Zabor's life are dreams and memories from which she draws clues for self-knowledge. In the process, she develops a viewpoint of what her whole life is about. This metaphoric process, Becker argues, is one avenue through which people attempt to create continuity following a period of disruption. Current events are then understood as part of tradition.

Nadia identifies a different point of intervention, related below in the form of three scenes. She does not focus on making sense of her life in Canada. She understands too well processes of margin-alization and exclusion. Her mission is to convey to the reader the structural violence (suffering) that she experiences—violence that arises from being deprived of the opportunity to work, which translates into lose of dignity and sense of self-worth. As noted above, the Canadian system "erased" Nadia's profession, leaving her no choice but to work in a dead-end part-time job in the social service sector. Having experienced this form of downward mobility to its lowest level, Nadia wanted to let the reader know that her becoming an oncologist—a rare profession for a woman—was a nuanced process. Nadia was keen to share her experiences on the larger struggles of her life, struggles that were informed by the discourse of modernity and gender. Nadia's starting point was her place of her birth: the first scene on the canvas of her life.

Scene One: Place of Birth
ജ

> I was born in a city called Riyat that is located in the [northern] part
> of Iran where the weather is very hot in summer and humidity is
> high too. This makes breathing extremely difficult as there is no air
> conditioner.

Descriptions of birthplaces serve as entry points into the lives of
people. Nadia's account suggests two readings. At one level she wants
to educate Canadian people on Iran, knowing full well that they
know next to nothing about this place, its way of life, its culture, its
literary traditions and its history—let alone the fine scholarship
produced by women over the last 150 years.[6] Nadia, like other Iranian
women, is concerned about the distorted images perpetuated by the
media, social service providers and also laypeople, the parameters
of which are as follows: Iranian people are uncivilized, backward
and oppressive to their women (the Orientalist discourse). In giving
a name to her place of birth, Nadia offers "a lesson in geography"—
a sense and a feel of where she is from. Simultaneously, she introduces
the reader to a second theme that on the surface refers to a lack: the
absence of air conditioners, which are a symbol of modernization.
It is important to note, however, that Nadia does not explain this
lack in terms of the Western master narrative of Iran's
"underdevelopment." She focuses on asymmetrical relations of
power, as evident in her further comment, "It is only in the oil
refineries where the Europeans worked that air conditioners were
available."

Nadia is well aware of the uneven state-initiated modernization
of Iran, through which the urban centres "benefitted" from the
modern infrastructure of schools, hospitals and communication
systems while the rural areas were not only bereft of these amenities
but were used to illustrate a contrasting image: "undeveloped" and
"backward." Middle East and Iranian feminist scholars have
emphasized the point that the state's project of modernizing has
never been free of ruptures, gaps and contradictions. Referring to
the literary campaign in rural Iran, Sullivan captures the irony of
tying village girls with the *chador* (outlawed by the Shah in 1934) to

prevent them from falling from English-style bunk beds in a boarding school:

> The image of the woman bound to her bed with the veil in the larger cause of progressive rights and freedoms, a paradox of modernity, captures the simultaneity of modernity and its underside, of the forces of reason and their bondage, of the necessary reconstruction of identity and the loss of community; it bears witness to modernity as its own gravedigger. (1998, 224)

As a woman from a rural area, Nadia was all too familiar with this contradictory trajectory. How she meandered her way through the emancipatory and regulatory impulses of modernity and gender is the theme that governs her account of "how I became a professional woman." In other words, what does it take for a woman to acquire the highest possible education in a situation where women are not accorded the full rights of a citizen except to serve the larger agenda of nationhood (Kandiyoti 1996, Abu-Lughod 1998)? By and large, woman and motherhood are conflated. In the case of Iran, women's identity is ideologically equated with the role of mothers, wives, daughters and sisters; *zan*, the Iranian term for a woman, is translated as "wife." However, this ideological stance contains multiple strands that are worthy of note.

There is no one point of entry into the subject of "gender," as this term—referred to as "the woman question"—encompasses a host of issues such as veiling and unveiling, family life, women's waged and non-waged work, polygamy and monogamy, sexuality and reproduction, women's culture and networks, and women's political and social activism (Keddie and Baron 1991, Abu-Lughod 1998, Nashat and Tucker 1999, Joseph and Slyomovics 2001). Friedl's research (1989, 1991) of two decades in an Iranian village is illustrative.

Friedl notes that women's everyday lives are hard to delineate. This is the case even in rural settings that "presumably offer relatively few roles and retain gender-role patterns longer than complex, fast-changing urban centres" (1991, 195). Women are said to belong in the house, "yet many women are out on legitimate errands for the whole day and far from home" (Ibid.,196). For Friedl, modernization has not worked in women's favour as it undermines women-centred networks and female solidarity. Furthermore, rural women's right to vote does not serve them well as decisions are made in distant urban centres; the same vote, this author argues, has taken away women's decision-making power that they exercised locally in pre-modern times when they had greater access to public spaces and sources of information.

Nadia's account of her mother's life also captures the complex phenomenon where women's designated space in the house (construed as confined and bound) was not the whole story. Consider Scene Two.

Scene Two: The World My Mother Gave Me
ೞ

Addressing the theme of a conference organized by the University of British Columbia on the subject of "The World My Mother Gave Me," Himani Bannerji observes that "our mothers are/were not in a position to give us much of the world, which mostly lay beyond their reach. Yet, they did leave us with an inheritance of a longing for the out-of-reach world" (2001, 2). Women's need to occupy a wider space of activity and movement in history, Bannerji notes, may be achieved through "lived moments of and through history, of women designing, rewriting their 'selves,' embodying the stories of being and becoming" (Ibid.).

In Iran, while Nadia was preparing herself for school and outside life, she does not dismiss her mother's interior world of home as insignificant. She considers it to have been an integral part of her story of being and becoming.

> My father used to work in the refinery company and my mother was a housewife and remained at home to take care of six children. She married my father when she was twelve years old and my father was forty years old at the time, a big age difference.

Nadia's pragmatic point of interjection into the popular discourse of early marriage (read: oppression) is worthy of note. She observes that her mother was an orphan and as such marriage gave her the opportunity to adopt the much-valorized roles of wife and mother as opposed to depending on her uncle for support. However, her mother became a widow at an early age:

> I was 12 years old when my father retired and my mother insisted that we move to another city, Quay. She insisted because she wanted to live close to her uncle, who at that time was living in Quay. We moved to Quay and after a month my father became ill and passed away. My 30-year-old mother was left with six young children and some savings at the bank and monthly pension of my father. We bought a house to live in and we had a simple condition of living. At that time I was in high school.

Nadia expressed admiration for her mother (an illiterate woman) for taking on the responsibility of raising six children (three daughters and three sons) on her husband's pension. She does not frame this event as something that her mother coped with in the absence of any other choice. She portrays her mother as someone who took charge of the house with realistic expectations that they were going to have "a simple condition of life." This observation draws our attention to the household as a unit of analysis in its own right. Only by doing so, as Hoodfar (1997) has argued, can we recognize women's economic behaviour.

Nadia's appreciation of her mother's resistance to what is commonly referred to as the "biomedical appropriation of women's bodies" is revealed in her retelling of how her mother refused to go to the nearby English hospital for the birth of her fourth child. The reason that she gave was "I did not want to leave my children alone." The broader context here is that of refusal to give up the home space, which, according to Nadia, was not confined to a mother/ father/children (nuclear family) unit, but opened up into more intricate areas. Nadia explained that the nature of these spaces cannot be easily described and needs to be experienced. During my brief visit to Iran (1999), I had the opportunity to participate in household activities in the cities of Tehran, Isfahan and Shiraz. I was struck by the array of issues that women discussed, ranging from women's rights to keeping abreast of developments abroad

(Iranian diaspora). Despite gender-segregation and forced re-veiling of women, I observed and was told that it is not a big deal for young adults (boys and girls) to party or swim in private pools. In fact, subversion of gender boundaries takes place on a daily basis.

There was a broader context to the decision made by Nadia's mother not to go to the hospital for the birth of her fourth child. We must note here that this is not an across-the-board stance, as women's use of the male-controlled health system may be governed by pragmatism (Lock and Kaufert 1998). Fahmy's (1998) example of Egypt is illustrative of the broader political context. Her research shows that the School of Midwives established by Mehmed Ali Pasha in the 19th century was ostensibly meant to "liberate" women. In reality, female doctors were given low positions from which they were expected to police other women's sexuality by verifying their virginity. For our purposes, it is important to note that Nadia does not present her mother, although illiterate, as being unaware of the way in which women are appropriated by the medical system.

Nadia shared a second example. In response to the Shah's 1936 decree of mass unveiling of women, Nadia's grandmother "went to the bathhouse at night with other women so that they would not be caught by the Shah's police." Her grandmother's refusal to unveil may be explained in relation to women's experiential knowledge that top-down approaches do not lead to fundamental changes. Milani brings to light a second dimension:

> This forced unveiling inflicted pain and terror upon those women who were not willing or ready to unveil. To them, the veil was a source of respect, virtue, protection and pride. It was a symbol of passage from childhood to adulthood .... They sought to undermine its banishment with all the ingenuity they could muster. (1992, 35)

The above examples reveal a subtext to "the world my mother gave me." Let us for a moment consider Afsaneh Najmabadi's insights. This Iranian scholar suggests that the project to educate women—an uneven project as attested by the urban-rural divide—formed part of the state agenda of building the nation. Women's education was promoted for two reasons: they would raise disciplined male citizens, and educated ("unveiled") women would help to subvert the Western colonial narrative of oppression of Middle Eastern women. The driving impulse for the former is this: "[F]rom educated women would arise a whole educated nation" (1998a, 102). Middle Eastern scholars have delineated the contours of the Western narrative as follows.

Middle Eastern scholars have argued that the West has created a particular kind of discourse where the East is conceived to be backward, inferior and frozen in time. This discourse, as Said (1978) argues, is entrenched institutionally so that the West comes to know about the Orient/the Other through scholarship, the media and through state policy. Images of women have been actively deployed in this narrative to further show the backwardness of the East. The argument advanced is to the effect that the barbaric nature of the East is revealed in the treatment it accords to its veiled and oppressed women. The script that is omitted is that of women in the West who continue to occupy subordinate positions despite feminist interventions (Ahmed 1992).

Iranian and Middle East male reformists undertook the task of countering Western discourse on Orientalism but failed to reverse gender discrimination. This is because their primary interest was to use women (materially, culturally, symbolically) for the purpose of nation-building. They were not in fact interested in "liberating" women.

In his work *Fatima Is Fatima*, Iranian writer Ali Shariati (1971) addresses two issues: to counter the "westoxicated" image of women that the Shah had promoted as an antidote to the West's perception of the East as backward, and to resolve the "problem of how women could enter modernity and remake themselves as neither western nor traditional" (cf. Sullivan 1998, 217). Shariati advocated women's rights for political ends. He advanced the argument that a woman who is excluded from literacy, education, culture and civilization cannot be expected to raise future generations that will build a nation. His reconfiguration of the image of Fatima is illustrative. Shariati de-emphasized Fatima's traditional image as the daughter of Prophet Muhammed, the wife of Imam Ali, and the mother of Hassan, Husain and Zainub (revered by Shi'a Muslims). He constructed a new image of Fatima as a woman who embodies revolutionary zeal—a quality desired at the time when the national struggle in Iran was both counter-monarchical and counter-Western. In another work, *One Followed by an Eternity of Zeros,* Shariati notes that Iran has fallen prey to "colonialism" that has denigrated Islam and Muslim women. The new gendered self then must be "a productive force in the service of nationalism deployed against the de-territorizing imperatives of western global capital" (cf. Sullivan 1998, 220).

Nadia's articulation with indigenous male discourses, as noted in the example provided by Shariati, is revealed in her account of education and work.

Scene Three: Occupying the Exterior/Interior Spaces
૪૭

I was able to pass the university exam and that was a big success for me. I went to the best university in Iran. It was a high-rank university in the Middle East. It was a good university and all the instruction was in English. That was the first time that I had to leave home and started my own life. It was a seven hour drive from my home city.

Nadia's birth in 1953 took place in the midst of major changes in the lives of Iranian women. The Shah's agenda of "catching up to the West" meant addressing "the woman's question"—a project undertaken by all nation-states. The Shah's attempts to emancipate women were half-hearted and the desired effect of transforming women's lives for the better never took root (Afkhami and Friedl 1994). In modern societies, women's emancipation in the way of education and waged work is filled with ambiguities. While they appear to have more opportunities in the public sphere, they are at the same time compelled to follow disciplinary routines, as illustrated in the case of Nadia (also see Abu-Lughod, 1988). While women were encouraged to obtain formal education and careers, it was for the purpose of rearing children "scientifically" and "rationally"—that is, raising disciplined citizens for the nation-state.

The above context suggests that the purpose of Nadia's university education cannot be reduced merely to the issue of her obtaining a career. Her schooling was part of the national agenda under which women's education was tied to the goal of raising good and disciplined citizens. As she relates her story of success and accomplishments, she also conveys that she felt the presence of the disciplinary life of regimentation ("the dark underside of modernity"). The regimentation included the lives of her children as well.

I worked hard and received a scholarship in the first year. In the second year, I applied for a student job at university and I got a job at a lab at my university. It was just enough for my food and other expenses. When I was in the fourth year of university I met my husband. After a few meetings, I figured out that he was the ideal man. After introducing him to my mother and my family, I got engaged. And we got married after two years. One year after, I gave birth to my daughter and 18 months later my son was born.

We moved to Tehran for continuing education and he [my husband] attended an engineering school and I attended a medical programme at my university. The university had a centre to look after the children of the staff and I was so lucky that I have a very nice place to put my children while I was at school. Every morning we had to take them to that centre and on my way back home in the afternoon, I picked them up. Come home, prepare meal and do cleaning and pack again for morning and got the kids to bed and then study till late night while the kids were sleeping. It was really hard. No complaint at all. I was working toward my goals. I finished school and then I got an excellent job at a university after a bit of competition and passing through the exams, interviews and all kinds of stuff. I was proud that I was the first in my family and also in my husband's family that a woman reach to that position. I enjoyed my work. I had a good reputation at the hospital and I did so well that I was promoted to a higher position just before I came to Canada.

My husband and I made our life. We worked hard, made money and buy a nice house and decorated it the way we would like. Of course it took us ten to eleven years to build it.

There is another aspect to Nadia's life and this concerns her attempts to remain socially connected to her natal home while attending university in Iran. It was only in my subsequent conversations that Nadia talked about her visits there. She stated that she and her family visited her mother's house weekly or biweekly. She described these visits and other special occasions (birthdays, New Year, Mother's Day) to be therapeutic in that they made her hard life at the university tolerable. Within the space of the home (which included her mother and her siblings, Nadia's siblings and their families, and also neighbours), Nadia experienced another mode of time, unstructured social time, captured in the work of the scholar Trinh T. Minh-ha:

> A mother continues to bathe her child amidst the group; two men go on playing a game they have started; a woman finishes braiding another woman's hair. These activities do not prevent their listening or intervening when necessary ... time and space are not something entirely exterior to oneself, something that one has, keeps, saves, wastes, or loses" (1989, 1–2).

Such visits are special. "Its (in)finitude subverts every notion of completeness and its frame remains a non-totalizable one," continues Trinh Minh-ha.

Nadia's visits to her home were a positive force in her life that circulated "like a gift; an empty gift which anybody can lay claim to by filling it to taste, yet can never truly possess. A gift built on multiplicity. One that stays inexhaustible within its own limits. Its departures and arrivals. Its quietness" (Ibid., 2).

Home as a site where social relationships are nurtured and knowledge of life acquired includes another dimension that has been subjugated and under-researched: the household economy that includes petty trade (selling items from home) and other female-centred activities. One of the few works that takes the household as an analytical unit for study comes from anthropologist Homa Hoodfar (1997). In her ethnographic research on low-income households in urban Egypt, this author notes how women and men respond to and cope with social and economic changes, including structural adjustment policies that downsize social service programmes to the detriment of ordinary people.

Working in rural areas in Iran and Egypt respectively, anthropologists Friedl (1991) and Abu-Lughod (1998) offer further insights on women's work and activities. Friedl's study shows how women (in southwest Iran) worked through and negotiated systems of power by subverting the private-public divide:

> [L]ocally, women are said to "belong in the house," yet one sees many women out on apparently legitimate errands, often all day and far from home ... a girl is taken out of school after the third grade because it is not right for her to be among strangers, but the next day she is working in an outpost camp in the mountains, in full view of women, men, relatives, and strangers alike. (Ibid., 196)

In her documentation of Awlad Ali Bedouin women, Abu-Lughod makes a case for same-sex socialization. She argues that this approach frees women from male surveillance and provides a milieu for raising children in a way that is not geared to them becoming future citizens of a proud nation. Women's roles as wives and mothers, she argues, are determined not through their dedication to their husbands or to the task of raising children but through their involvement with the affairs of their kin and women's community. A significant issue highlighted here is the blurring of boundaries between the public and the private. Women's work in the kin-based arena is as public as men's work "outside the home." In the light of this research, Abu-Lughod critiques gender-based reforms advocated by Amin on the grounds that they were geared towards producing "good bourgeois wives and mothers in a world where state and class ties would override those of kin, capitalist organization would divide the world into distinct sphere of private and public, and women would be subjected to husbands and children, cut off from their kin and other women" (1998, 261).

Nadia's home visits, which embody the contradictions of modernity, as noted above, may be read in the context of women's desire to keep alive their experiential knowledge acquired through kin-based interactions. These "story times" are created by women themselves out of elements that are both new and old. Within the framework of non-linear time, they air issues and exchange new information on such diverse topics as a relative's visit abroad, a health issue, women's economic activities and so on.

In the above section we have looked at two sets of data: the so-called emancipatory discourses of writers such as Ali Shariati, and ethnographic studies that portray women's agency shaped by particular social, historical and political situations.

Studies of women living in urban centres along the lines discussed above are scarce. The literature presents urban women as engulfed by the market sphere and their home lives are barely mentioned except in terms of their double load. The complexities and nuances captured in the studies of women in rural areas in Iran and elsewhere in the Middle East *appear* not to exist in the urban landscape, but clearly this is a false assumption. With this in mind, I have endeavoured to include Nadia's account of her home visits, which she did not elaborate upon but considered to be vital. Her unwillingness to talk about this part of life may be due to the fact that a "vocabulary" adequate for talking about women's lives in the domestic sphere has not been sufficiently developed, as Devault (1990) has rightly observed.

In her narrative, Nadia presents herself as a person who has worked through the larger discourse on modernity and gender. Her profile of her career life includes lives of her mother and grandmother, and her home visits. While this may appear ordinary, there is a layered context in place—the context being that Nadia's life constitutes part of the gendered discourse on modernity and nationhood. In her new homeland in Canada, this discourse has not even assumed a faint shape: immigrant women's lives do not form part of the social and national imagination of the state.

In this chapter, I have shown that the race/gender/class paradigm does not tell the full story: it omits agency. The second paradigm of civil/small voices brings to light a nuanced context that reveals that Nadia's life, like those of her cohort, encompasses larger issues. From this point of view, Nadia's resettlement in Canada led not only to the erasure of her professional life but also to the nuances and contexts of the larger project of modernity and gender where Nadia was an active player. This denuding of struggle and meaning had a direct bearing on Nadia's mental health and well-being.

Conclusion

ℬ

My response to Nadia's question "Why is it hard for a professional immigrant woman to find work in Canada?" has prompted me to address the tension between the paradigms of intersectionality (race/gender/class) and civil/small voices. The former has brought into relief the channelling of the majority of immigrant women into low-paying jobs. Here we may note that legislative attempts to remedy gender inequalities in Canada—the *Employment Equity Act*/Bill C62—does not substantively include women of colour in comparison to "visible minority" men and white women (Boyd 1992). Nadia's story reveals the process through which women of colour are excluded from professional work. As we noted, Nadia's search for work in her area of expertise thrust her into a ghettoized dead-end job. This is the state agenda that counts on the cheap labour of immigrant women to fill in the gaps created by the downsizing of the social service sector. The state also works towards keeping immigrant women in their place as they are not expected to "fill the professional social space, but that of manual and industrial labour or the lower levels of white collar jobs" (Bannerji 1995, 134). As has been well noted, racialized women continue to fuel the ghettoized global market economy (Ong 1987, Mohanty 2003).

In relating her experiences of structural exclusion (read: suffering), Nadia tells a second story of modernity and gender as it unfolds in her country of origin. This second story is explicated by Abu-Lughod with reference to three points. First is the incorporation of women into the political agenda of the nation-state and global capitalism, which may be understood at two levels: discursive and material. The discursive level comes into play in the way in which women and their bodies (veiling/unveiling, for example) "have become potent symbols of identity and visions of society and the nation" (1998, 3). Materially, non-Western women's low-paid work advances capitalist interests, nationally and globally (Mohanty 2003, Harrison 1997). Second is women's own participation in the project on modernity and gender in relation to how they manoeuvre and work thorough the contradictions that engulf their lives. Nadia's narrative on how she became an oncologist illustrates this point further: modernity for her was liberating but also constraining in the way in which it individualized her—in her country of resettlement she had to wage her battles alone, away from her husband and in the absence of the kind of female-centred networks that she had nurtured in her country of birth. The third dimension concerns the imperialist narrative on the oppressed Muslim women. This narrative, as Middle East scholars (Fahmy 1998, Keddie 1991, Najmabadi 1998) have noted, serves to advance the image of the West as saviour of Muslim women. Here, we may note that the response of Islamic states has not worked in favour of women. As the Iranian scholar Sullivan has expressed it:

> In Iran's conflicted efforts to construct national, revolutionary, and Islamic modernities the figure of the "woman" has repeatedly been constituted as the overdetermined sign of an essentialized totality, as a metaphor for a besieged nation, an embattled self, a delicate interiority, the uncontrollable other, the "unpierced pearl" to be bought and protected, or the sacred interior. (1998, 228)

The particular status accorded to women is encapsulated in the symbol of the veil. As noted earlier, the Shah's alliance with the West led to forced unveiling of women while the anti-Western stance of the Islamic Republic of Iran led to the re-veiling of women. In Milani's words, "Forcefully unveiled, they personify the modernization of the nation. Compulsorily veiled, they embody the reinstitution of the Islamic order" (cf. Sullivan, Ibid., 228).

The three points of women as potent symbols of identity for society, women as active agents in the discourse on gender and modernity, and the Western script on gender politics—all are encapsulated in Nadia's narrative. The discursive and material appropriation of immigrant women's bodies—the race/class/gender paradigm—helps us to understand why Nadia is not able to find work in her area of expertise. However, this is not the end point for Nadia. Exercising agency, she introduces the reader to the wider arena where modernity as a gendered project (Abu-Lughod's framework) is profiled on "the canvas of life" discussed above. The "scenes" in the canvas exemplify the ambiguous project of modernity as being both emancipatory and constraining for women. Nadia's acquisition of professional education was a negotiated process unfolding on the canvas of "the dark underside of modernity" (Abu-Lughod, 1998) as well as within the more positive, open spaces of home (natal and marital). In crossing the border with this complex small-voices story, Nadia subverts the colonial/Western narrative of Muslim women as backward and oppressed.

The analytical framework of the two paradigms has allowed us to move beyond the reification of the text into the making of the text where the presence of gendered agency becomes manifest. At this level we can "talk about women as historical subjects and in terms of their historical experiences" (Ong 1987, xiii). The emphasis on gendered agency points to the fact that the most important form of action take place at the margins—among the civil/small voices. As Ortner (1994, 391) has aptly expressed it: it is these forms of action that brings into relief the shape of any given system. This aspect was brought home to me during our last meeting when Nadia said: "When I first came to Canada, I was full of hopes and dreams. I had worked hard in Iran and I was willing to do that here too. Now I have just stopped dreaming. I have stopped trying." Not having a space to express her agency in her new homeland, Nadia resorts to telling her story through the civil/small voices paradigm to ensure that she is not cast as a victim.

Insights from the two paradigms position us to give a politicized and humane (not faceless) response to Nadia's question as to why she, and other immigrant women, are not able to work in their areas of expertise in Canada. Between the spaces of the two paradigms we can vigorously interrogate and challenge the exclusionary practices of the Canadian labour force and the gendered project of modernity where women continue to find themselves on the margins. It is from these very spaces that women tell their stories of suffering to effect change.

Notes

1   The committee focused on identifying cultural differences. Political economy of health has not made inroads into service organizations or the health care system.

2   In her search for work in her area of expertise, it was logical for Nadia to join a health committee. She was soon to discover that the only kind of "work" available for her

was voluntary. Downsized health sector counts on unemployed and partially employed women to fill the gaps left by the state.

3   I cite these examples to pay tribute to the authors for their fine analysis. Also, these examples represent a larger body of work that falls under the rubric of political economy.

4   Nadia's marginal status as a displaced racialized woman gives her cause for reflection articulated through the telling of herstory.

5   Names of people, places and occupations have been changed to protect the privacy of the research participants. Other changes have been made to accommodate Nadia's suggestions on confidentiality.

6   This is true. My field research revealed that mainstream people know very little about the rich heritage and culture of Iran. During the mall-walking programme, some elderly white women posed such questions as whether it snowed in Iran or if Iranian people had refrigerators.

FIVE

Between Speech and Silence:
Sahra's Story

I was somebody once. I had a huge house in Iran. Here, in Canada, I am living in a tiny apartment that does not even have space to put my shoes.

I am not the type to depend on the children.

The desire that I have is to one day revisit my great homeland in Iran, and encounter a new and improved Iran, where people can live with their differences in peace and harmony.

What I have presented above are extracts of a narrative that Sahra, a 70-year-old woman, dictated to her daughter Rima over a course of three months in 1999. I "met" Sahra and her daughter at a well-being session that the ESL Iranian coordinator had organized in response to my suggestion for a forum on storytelling.[1] The coordinator, in conjunction with other Iranian women, used the forum to test the feasibility of a pilot project on well-being. Her intent was to convince a funding agency of the therapeutic value of storytelling, otherwise dismissed as a leisurely pursuit.[2]

Researchers (Frank 2000, Ong 1995a) have noted the creative and politicized use of field situations by research participants. Sahra had her own take on the situation. She chose her daughter (grandson on another occasion) as a person who would cross the border with her story. This border is best considered as fluid so as to facilitate the telling and retelling of her story to multiple audiences: her family members who had only heard Sahra's story in bits and pieces; participants of the storytelling session where Sahra's story resonated with that of another woman—"I have nothing to live for. When I get up in the morning I am sad and depressed. When I go to bed, I am in the same state"[3]—the researcher/reader; the two service providers who attended the session; and the teacher who heard Sahra's story through her grandson's school project. In choosing to tell her story of pain and suffering to her daughter, Sahra wished to record her life for posterity. The desire to undertake such an activity is especially strong among people whose lives have been rendered socially invisible (Good 1994, Myerhoff 1978).[4]

In taking the leap towards producing her own text, Sahra reversed the power dynamics in the field, much like Gelya Frank's (2000) research subject who introduced Frank as "my biographer" and not as "my researcher." It is important to recognize the initiative that the research participants take to express their agency and create themselves as subjects. The researchers' assumption that they have the sole "power" to create space for the participants to speak reintroduces power dynamics through the back door. Sahra's narrative carries the issue of voice a step further and poses a challenge to the reader: Do we merely record stories of pain and suffering or should we engage in the act of witnessing? If the latter, how do we go about doing this?

A response to the above questions calls for a departure from conventional modes that focus on words as the only source of reading and interpreting a story. In this chapter, I argue that sufferers use silence as the language of communication and that validating this mode of expression is a first step towards taking the leap from being a detached observer to a vulnerable and witnessing one. Examples from the literature along with a chronological reading of Sahra's text will elucidate this point further. The latter is in keeping with the way Sahra frames her story: childhood years, adulthood, and old age. In a concluding note, I comment on the dynamic relationship between silence and speech.

The Act of Witnessing

ఐ

In *Vulnerable Observer*, anthropologist Ruth Behar (1996) describes an example of witnessing. Behar portrays a fictive scenario of a photographer, Rolf Carle, who records and casts his gaze on a 13-year-old girl trapped in the 1985 avalanche in Colombia. As the girl's heart and lung collapse, Rolf Carle crouches down in the mud and throws his arms around the girl.

Behar uses this scenario to pose a number of questions: How can we connect with our ethnographic participants without Othering them? Is it possible for an ethnographer to do both: engage in the act of self-exposure and be a spectator? Do we act to release another from suffering or do we simply observe? The issues raised here continue to engage the attention of anthropologists because the ethics of our discipline, according to Behar, do not always allow us to represent what we see and hear in the field. What Behar does not take into account is that the ethnographic participants may also engage anthropologists on these very issues. By authoring her own text and using the silence-and-speech medium of communication, Sahra also responds to the questions posed by Behar. Let us look at some examples from the literature.

My first example comes from Fiona Ross's work on "The Hearings of the South African Truth and Reconciliation Commission." Taking a gendered perspective, this author argues that we must learn to read silence in women's testimonies. Like Visweswaran (1994), she recognizes that women's subordinate social position does not allow them to tell in words their stories of pain and suffering. Ross, however, cautions us not to impute silence as a marker of passivity. She argues that silence is women's signature of agency as it is through this medium of communication that women convey layers of experiences that are dismissed in official narratives. Her analysis of women's testimonial data indicates that women speak in a rich language, using socially valorized metaphors such as those of family and domesticity. "The emphasis on domestic context in women's stories highlights the failures of home to protect and contain, and points to state intrusion at many levels. The specificity with which women detailed their domestic worlds and time points to the depths of state irruption in them" (Ross 2001, 268). The listener's task, she concludes, is to acknowledge that silence marks particular kinds of knowing and that "women's silences can be recognized as language, and we need carefully to probe the cadences of silences, the gaps between fragile words, in order to hear what women say" (2001, 273).

On a second front, Maya Todeschini's research on the bombed Japanese women (Hiroshima and Nagasaki 1945) reveals that subordinate groups await appropriate time and context before speaking; otherwise they risk the possibility of not being heard. In the case of Japanese women, this author shows that they could only speak and subvert the official narrative on bombing—narrative that had dismissed their lived reality as inconsequential—when they assumed the culturally recognized status of motherhood. In their stories, the bombed women (*hibakusha* women) avoided using the official discourse that subdued their experiences. Using the metaphor of the body as a weapon, the women conveyed the message that they were the embodiment of radiation—a position that subverted the official narratives that de-legitimized their anxieties concerning their disrupted roles of social and biological producers of human species. Women's discourse on the embodiment of the bomb allowed them to invoke a gendered vulnerability through which they could transform "their tainted bodies, the fear of producing abnormal offspring, into a weapon to reclaim the bomb as a moral and ethical issue that concerns the community as a whole" (2001, 137).

So far we have established that the act of witnessing and listening to silence involves two impulses: (a) to assume the position of a vulnerable observer blurring the conventional boundaries of objectivity and subjectivity to the extent possible, and (b) to listen to the silences between words in order to establish a context for a richer and a fuller story, thereby validating experiences of pain and suffering that otherwise remain unrecognized. Once we acknowledge that women's silence can be recognized as language, we can engage in more layered reading of the text in question. The genre of silence lends itself to three performative acts: retrieval of voice, a first step towards healing; testimonial speaking, where one voice represents a polyphony of other voices; and women's use of metaphors and words, through which they establish their moral authority. We may note here that the language of silence creates a collective identity and a bond among women. Women can then witness each other's stories of pain and suffering.

In the light of the above, the Iranian storytelling session may be read as an act of witnessing; here women read the silences between words and also continued where others had stopped without bringing a closure to their stories. The women were also engaged in presenting a collective front so that "one woman's story was everyone's story" in the way of testimonial speaking.

The above examples show that subordinate groups use multiple mediums to convey their experiences of pain and suffering. Among these mediums, silence is an important marker of agency. Silence does not rule out speech. Once we acknowledge that women's silence can be recognized as language, we can learn to read "the cadences of silences, the gaps between fragile words, in order to hear what it is that women say," to reiterate Ross's important observation.

We have also noted that silence is not confined to a lone voice but gives rise to a collective identity: "Black women of the apartheid era" and "the bombed women of Hiroshima and Nagasaki." A collective front makes it possible for women to speak authoritatively about their condition as a whole, with all its contradictions and nuances. Sahra's sharing of her story, as noted earlier, was not an isolated occurrence. She was motivated to speak at a time when other Iranian women were telling their stories to each other in the presence of service providers and the researcher.

A common theme of displacement and well-being (read: pain and suffering/the soft knife of politics) informed the women's stories, despite variations in relation to particular trajectories of life. It must be noted that, ironically, women's most intense experiences of pain were felt in Canada, the place where they had sought refuge. As one woman expressed it: "It was easier to live in turmoil back at home because we did not expect anything different. But here in Canada, we were not prepared for this kind of suffering and hardship."

The experiences of suffering concern isolation and lack of opportunity for work and social engagement. This situation, as noted earlier, was brought about by structural exclusion of Iranian women from the nation-state of Canada, along with their social construction as the Other. Structural exclusion and Othering has been an integral part of Sahra's life, first in Iran, then as a refugee in El Salvador and Japan, and finally as a landed immigrant in Canada. Sahra's sharing of her story then is directed towards evoking a response from the reader/listener. Sentiments like those expressed by Sahra are captured by Arthur Frank:

> The ill, and all those who suffer, can also be healers. Their injuries become the source of the potency of their stories. Through their stories, the ill create empathic bonds between themselves and their listeners. These bonds expand as the stories are retold. Those who listen tell others, and the circle of shared experience widens. Because stories can heal, the wounded healer and wounded storyteller are not separate but are different aspects of the same figure. (1995, xii)

Reading Sahra's Story
ও

The story I now present follows a different set of narrative conventions. Sahra's testimony highlights the language of the body that evokes social and political contexts in ways that resonate with stories of other Iranian women. Sahra then speaks to layers of experiences entwined in a wide set of social relations. Hidden in her story are forms of knowledge and agency that need to be validated and sensitively heard.

ও Early Years of Life: Childhood and Marriage

"I was born into a family who lived in the centre of Iran in a dry hot desert city called Yazd. Not only were the temperature uncomfortable and at times unbearable, so were the people." By putting people and harsh desert climate on the same plane, Sahra conveys with intensity the persecution of the Baha'i community, and the sense of mission that governed her early life. As a second daughter in the family, Sahra was compelled to deal with social oppression with the help of her father, whom she considered to be a "very capable, strong man. He had undying faith that carried him through hard times." Her mother was caring but naïve and also sick, as Sahra put it: "From the time I can remember, my mother was always ill." It then fell upon Sahra to perform household tasks from a young age.

> At the age of five, I would do the shopping for the entire household while also caring out the duties of vacuuming and cleaning the home on a regular basis. A few years after this time, at the age of ten, I was looking after and caring for my six younger siblings.

It is interesting to note that Sahra makes no mention of the role that her elder sister and other older siblings would have played in running the house. This silence may be explained in relation to two factors. First, Sahra's story is a testimonial that as a matter of fact captures a poignant loss: namely, loss of childhood brought about by a political situation, the everyday impact of which included remembering "my father coming home after receiving beatings in the street." Second, first-person talk/silence allows Sahra to speak with authority, as in her comment that "I have been there and so you have to believe my story."

As Frank has expressed it: "In stories, the teller not only recovers her voice; she becomes a witness to the conditions that rob others of their voices. When any person recovers her voice, many people begin to speak through that story" (1995, xii). Sahra beckons us to listen through the cadences of silence in her story. This message is brought home through her vivid accounts of two other events: martyrdom and marriage.

Martyrdom

Sahra's account of martyrdom begins at the time her father was 2 years old: "He was forced to endure a great hardship. My grandfather, who was his father, was martyred simply for his belief in a religion, the Baha'i faith." On her mother's side, there were seventeen religious martyrdoms. It is difficult for us to imagine what it is like to lose eighteen members in one family. Sahra takes the reader into the heart of everyday life where the impact of tragedy is keenly felt. She recalls how her mother would sit by the door around 4 p.m. listening for her husband's footsteps. If her mother heard the sound of wobbling, she would run out with her first-aid kit to bandage the wounds he suffered from beatings he received on his way home. Sahra recalled how her family was forced to forgo sleep so that they could draw water at night from the well—a source that they were forbidden to use. On the other hand, Sahra also related "acts of kindness" when Muslims would sell them bread under the table and would look the other way when the Baha'is would touch the fruit on the stalls. During times when no Baha'i was to be hired by a Muslim, some prospective employers changed the names on the forms to prevent the employee's detection by the state. Baha'is could accept this, but, according to Sahra, would never write their own names differently "so firm were they in their beliefs." Referring to her father's life, Sahra notes:

> Due to the untimely death of my grandfather, my father was forced to accept the responsibility of caring for his two sisters and his mom for most of his life. Although the situation was brought upon his shoulders, he graciously accepted it, and his strong character enabled him to do a fine job.

Soon after, another tragedy hit the family. Her aunt's husband died in a car accident. This time her father took charge of eight of his children.

> Now my father would look after not only his two sisters and his mother along his own wife and children, but he would also become the father to his eight nephews and nieces. My responsibility became much greater as well, as I would also have to watch over my cousins.

People who go through difficult times feel the need to tell their stories to recover their voice, which pain and suffering have taken away. But the voice that speaks also (re)members how disrupted events are reconstituted so that life can go on even under the most difficult circumstances. As the sufferer recovers her voice, other people can speak through the story that is being related. Through recovering her voice (the act of storytelling), Sahra becomes a witness to the collective experiences of her family. In a situation of pain and suffering, many people can speak through the story of one person.

This explains why Sahra once again does not bring up the role of her siblings in the enormous amount of care and work that now formed part of her familial life.

Marriage

> At a mere fifteen years of age, I married a 25-year-old man. It was not arranged, as were the majority of the weddings at the time. Rather it was two people who genuinely fell in love.

Sahra considers her marriage as compensation for her difficult childhood experiences. Her happiness was enhanced by the fact that her husband's family was well-to-do and that her mother-in-law loved her like a daughter. But this state of affairs did not last for long, as once again her life was encompassed by struggles for survival. Her family was hit by a cycle of bankruptcies.

> My husband's family business went bankrupt. He had ran the business with his father and his brother, and at this point, his father would stay at home while his brother made every attempt to revive the business and bring it out of bankruptcy.

To assist the family, Sahra's husband (Riaz) took on the job of a teacher, a position that compelled him to be on the move—being sent from one village to another—"just because he was a Baha'i." This and many other state-initiated strategies were put into place to make life difficult for members of the Baha'i community. Sahra stated that she survived the family bankruptcies partly because of the happiness she felt at the birth of her children. "At the same time [as the bankruptcy] my first daughter was born. The joy of this birth would come to balance the sorrow of the bankruptcy." Her husband joined the family business once it was revived, but not for long.

> After a while, my first son was born, and along with his birth came the second bankruptcy of the business. This time around, the bankruptcy hit hard, and shocked and saddened everyone involved. My husband went back to teaching. This time around, he was destined to be the "travelling" teacher ....

By the time Sahra was 22 years old, she had four children (two boys and two girls) and had moved nine times with her husband. Then came a cathartic event that made Sahra speak through her wounds: her 4-year-old son accidentally swallowed a coin. "The coin remained in his body and when the doctors tried to remove it in the small town we were living in, they were unsuccessful. Not only did they fail but they actually did more damage to his body [liver]." Sahra and her husband took their son to Tehran for treatment, a move that compelled Riaz to leave his work. Sahra's family in Yazd took care of the other children.

The treatment took six months, during which time the family stayed with acquaintances. "Since we would not dare be a burden to any of these families, we would constantly be on the move with a very sick child to make our stay pleasant with each household." But her son's condition got worse. The coin was removed with ease but the wounds on the liver could not be healed. At the house where Sahra was staying at that time, the woman had become pregnant after three miscarriages. Her husband and family members were trying to ensure that she was not exposed to bad news of any kind.

> On my son's last surgery, it became evident that he only had a short time to live as the doctors could not do anything more to help. On the night that he passed away, my husband and I alerted no one so as to not upset the fragile lady of the home. I buried my face into a pillow and cried all through the night so she would not hear my sorrow. In the morning, I carried the dead body of my son covered in a blanket and without informing them of the tragedy, thanked them and walked away as if nothing was wrong and my child was merely sleeping.

When Sahra returned to Yazd she had to console her two older children, "who had grown to dearly love their younger brother," and she had to bond with her 1-year-old daughter. She did not mourn in front of the children "so as not to upset them any further .... I held back my tears for months. It is only natural for a mother to have to mourn her child and in order to do that, visible signs of emotion are necessary. For me to have to deny this was incredibly difficult." She continues:

All this stress came symbolically to a halt one day a few months after the passing of my son. I had decided to go to the storage area to do some cleaning and while I was doing this, I came across some of my son's clothing from the time he was a baby. Nothing would stop me at this point as the tears began to flow continuously. These were my first tears in many months and with the children not around, I didn't hold myself back. Right after this I got very sick with rheumatism and after four months this disease affected me greatly to the point that I could barely walk.

Sahra did not openly mourn the death of her son in order that another woman could have "peace"; Sahra did not openly mourn the death of her son in order that her children would be spared the grief. Sahra is the sacrificial mother who swallows pain so that other people's lives are not disrupted. But the script does not end here. In embodying (swallowing) pain that should otherwise have been shared, Sahra effects a spatial shift from the individual to the social. This is because when the body speaks it implicates society. As Frank has expressed it, the body is not mute, it is inarticulate: "it does not use speech, yet begets it ..." (1995, 2). When the body is not medicalized (read: individualized), it reveals societal fault lines. The fault line in question is continual marginalization of the Baha'i community from the nation-state of Iran.

Sahra's inability to mourn for her son is correlated to this structural factor. Her collapsed body ("I could barely walk") is a commentary on the treatment that Iranian society accorded to her, her family and her community. Sahra's body language (the language of silence) announces the lifelong hardships (socially incurred) that she and her family endured as members of the Baha'i community. A summary statement on the Baha'is would be helpful.

ಇ The Community

The Baha'i religion was founded in Iran in the mid-19th century under the leadership of Bab. Bab claimed that he was both the prophet of a new revelation and the twelfth Imam whose return was expected by the Shi'as, the religion of the majority in Iran. The Iranian clerical establishment thus perceived the Baha'i faith as a threat to their status and power. It is not surprising that during times of political instability, the persecution of the Baha'is reached its height, leading to execution of its leaders. The Baha'is do not enjoy the civil rights accorded to the citizens of Iran. Compared with other religious minorities such as the Jews, the Christians and the Zoroastrians, the Baha'is fare worse (Baha'i International Community 1981, Taherzadeh 1992). Depending on the political agendas of the people in power, the Baha'is have been denied employment and opportunities for higher education. Their property has been confiscated and the community as a whole has been subject to continual physical and verbal harassment. Yet, the Baha'is have persevered despite tremendous odds, including mass execution of their leaders. Social oppression and centuries of persecution have resulted in one development in which the Baha'is take pride: they are a well-educated community spread around the world (Kazemzadeh 2000).

The elements noted above are reflected in Sahra's life story. She considers her family as pioneers of the faith, but this status has meant sacrifice on her part. She embodies her family's pain and suffering, as noted above. It is her wound then that tells her story and that of her family and community.

Political Subjectivity

ഇ

In her work on *nervos*/hunger among the people of Alto do Cruzeiro (Brazil), Nancy Scheper-Hughes advances two possibilities. On the one hand, a person "can be open and responsive to the covert language of the organs, recognizing in his trembling hands and 'paralyzed' legs the language of suffering, protest, defiance, and resistance." On the other hand, "he can silence it, cut it off by surrendering more and more of his consciousness and pain to the technical domain of medicine, where they will be transformed into a 'disease' to be treated with an injection, a nerve pill, a soporific. Once safely medicated, however, the scream of protest is silenced, and the desperate message in the battle is lost" (1992, 214).

Sahra's narrative reveals that the language of the body, however subdued, is never silenced. The issue is whether we can develop the sensibility to hear the story emanating from the body. The circumstances of Sahra's life determined her use of body language and the language of silence.

The storage incident, Sahra informs us, made her feel better despite the fact that the family had to make a fresh start: "We lost all of our money once again and had to borrow a loan to start our life [from the] ground up once again." Eight years after the death of her son, "we were in happy times once again: my last child, a beautiful girl, was born, bringing happiness to everyone in the family." Once again, however, their happiness was short-lived.

Faced by ongoing persecution, many Baha'is, including Sahra's three older children, left Yazd. Settling in three different countries (El Salvador, Philippines and Germany), each child acted as a pioneer of the Baha'i faith. Sahra and her family (husband and 10-year-old daughter) moved to Tehran. Sahra's husband secured a good job and the couple bought a big house. "Our new house was massive, but seemed so empty without the entire family." Sahra did not have much time to think of the vacuum left by the absence of her children. The new Islamic government did not take kindly to the Baha'i community. Sahra expresses her distress using body language (describing symptoms):

> I suffered a major car accident around this time in Iran. I was lucky to be alive, and was in crutches and a body in cast for one year. Even up to this day, when specific parts of my body are lightly touched, I feel great pain.

Medical anthropologists have informed us that the body in sickness is a "polysemic system" (Lock and Kaufert 1998, 16). Consider the observations made by French:

> [E]ven the most apparently subjective and personal of experiences—the experience of one's own body—is shaped in important ways by the relations of power and domination in which the body is involved. These relationships are embedded in the social order and part of the experience of everyone who participates in that order. (1994, 69)

The fact that Sahra places the accident between a personal/familial occurrence (settling down in Tehran) and a highly charged political event (forced migration out of the country), cautions us not to confine ourselves to a discreet reading of this event. Our attention is drawn to a body in cast, a body in pain. This body implicates the social. A body in cast exists in a disengaged state from the world but ironically it is in this immobilized state that it gains power to speak. As the individual body exists "as a social hieroglyph in mythic communication with others," to use Allen Feldman's words (cf. French, Ibid.), what it has to say must be contextualized. In Sahra's case the context concerns momentary withdrawal (one year) from a society that has not been kind to her. A body in pain continues to engage the world in a manner that critiques and identifies the societal fault lines as much as do the hungry bodies of the people of Alto in northeast Brazil (Scheper-Hughes 1992). This framework of analysis informs Sahra's narrative of migration and re-settlement in Canada in her advanced years.

❧ Forced Migration and Settlement

Nation-states are fragile units whose socially constructed boundaries are permeable and subject to perceived symbolic and military threats. The fragility of the nation-state is a function of its elitist and exclusive make-up (Lee and Cardinal 1998). Minorities (including women) are then policed and contained to ensure that they do not disrupt the status quo of this imagined unit; the policing is accentuated during uncertain times such as revolution or economic crisis. The persecution of the Baha'i community may be explained within this framework. As an indigenous movement (1840s) within Shi'a Islam, the Baha'is have been considered to be a particular threat. During the time of the Iranian Revolution, in Sahra's words,

> The Baha'is were being bothered and discriminated against at an alarming rate. The wealthier Baha'is, who were the main target of the uprising, left Iran. The revolution of Iran was about to begin. The Shah of Iran was ousted and things were getting dangerous. The Islamic Republic of Iran was established, and with the establishment, the Baha'is were being arrested or killed for nothing except their belief. The stress that seemed to disappear in the past few years all rushed back tenfold .... The one aspect of their attack that frightened me the most was the way they would target young girls.

These circumstances compelled Sahra to send her 13-year-old daughter to a Baha'i school in India, a step that was difficult for Sahra as she felt lonely without her children. When Sahra got the news that five members of her husband's religious committee had been arrested and martyred, she decided to leave Iran. Sahra's observations are echoed by Farr (1999), who notes that soon after the Revolution, many Baha'is were attacked by angry mobs. Out of the 700 Baha'i leaders who were detained, many were killed. Under these circumstances, Sahra's husband, Riaz, got 400,000 *tomans* (Iranian currency) for a house that had cost him 2 million *tomans*, and his retirement money was cut off.

> Everything that we had come to know was suddenly gone from our very eyes. With nothing but two suitcases, we left for El Salvador where my son was living. When we left the country we didn't realize that we would be leaving for good. All my dreams were violently shattered.

In El Salvador, Sahra and her husband started a new life.

> [M]y husband was able to get some work. He would be a baker in our own house (with a lot of my help), and we would approach various stores and sell the sweets at a bulk. We once again started from the ground up, and didn't do so poorly.

Sahra stated that she felt depressed owing to "the sudden departure from home I had known for the longest time ...." Her youngest daughter from India joined them and registered for a course in dentistry. Soon after, there was a revolution in El Salvador and the family was compelled to leave for Japan. As refugees they feared for their safety.

In Japan, Sahra and Riaz experienced cultural shock as they did not know the language and "we were not used to the food and their culture is one of the most unique in the entire world." With the little money that they had, and drawing upon their experience in El Salvador, the couple started a bakery business, but it did not work "as the idea of selling sweets out of your own home wasn't such a success with the Japanese and we lost all our money that we had invested. We were bankrupt once again." Her husband retired because there was no work for him in their adopted country, and this meant that the couple had to turn to their daughter and son-in-law for financial support. The fact that her 63-year-old husband had to stay at home was hard for Sahra: "[I]t crushed him and it hurt me to have to watch him suffer internally."

While in Japan, Sahra, then in her early fifties, got the news that her eldest daughter's seventeen-year marriage was coming to an end. All the sisters kept the news away from her because of her fragile health. Eventually, they let her know:

When it became official, there was no choice but for my daughters to tell me. This news broke my spirit and I got ulcers and my stomach began to bleed internally. I needed an operation, and after this operation, two-thirds of my stomach had been removed. Soon after, her second daughter who had been married for a short time to her cousin was divorced. A third incident concerned the death of her daughter-in-law from cancer. For Sahra the cumulative impact of these crises was: "I was my weakest, illest [sic], most unstable point.

During this time, an earthquake occurred in Kobe. Once again, Sahra resorts to body language:

Physically and emotionally at an all-time low, we moved to Canada. Since my diabetes was related to stress, and I was immensely stressed out, my diabetes had become unmanageable. Due to the earthquake I was emotionally traumatized. Again I was forced to leave with my daughter (who had migrated to Canada from Japan six months before the earthquake). The idea of me burdening my daughter was hard to handle. I began to lose weight and became quite sick.

The fact that her lifetime struggle, perseverance and hard work were giving way to a state of dependency was unbearable for Sahra. She experienced depression that resonated with that of another woman in the storytelling session, as noted above. "When I get up in the morning, I am sad and depressed. When I go to bed, I am in the same state." As for her life in Canada, Sahra did not have much to say except "My house does not have enough room for my own shoes." This sentence is emblematic of the physical and social confinement that has been Sahra's experience as an aging immigrant woman in Canada. Her concerns were articulated through the silent language of the body.

The Silent Language of the Body
❧

"People certainly talk about their bodies in illness stories; what is harder to hear in the story is the body creating the person," writes A. Frank (1995, 53). Body begets speech at the time when language fails. How do we then recognize a speaking body? In other words, how do we witness a bodily-inscribed story? The literature suggests two approaches.

Representing the first approach, Arthur Kleinman (1988) suggests that the body speaks through symptoms of illness. Bodily expressions of symptoms, he argues, contain two messages: (a) embodiment of social trauma, and (b) transformative possibilities, also referred to as bodily praxis (Lock and Kaufert 1998). Note that this latter process does not occur as a matter of course. Lived bodies create history and it is within this space that the body expresses itself socially. Hence, it is through the language of symptoms that the speaking body endeavours to connect with the world.

Arthur Frank's work exemplifies the second approach. This author notes that bodies are communicative by nature and hence they use stories to convey critical messages to the world. Rather than being individual acts of narration, the stories, notes Frank, contain narrative truths suppressed by the dominant language. Stories make it possible for sufferers to position themselves as witnesses to their traumas, inviting audiences to reciprocate by becoming witnesses in turn. This is what gives the story its power.

As Frank expresses it, "What makes an illness story good is the act of witnessing that says, implicitly or explicitly, 'I will tell you not what you want to hear but what I know to be true because I have lived it'" (1995, 63). For Frank, reclaiming of a voice begins with the body, which creates the self that connects with people who empathize with the sufferer. In this context we can understand the observation made by the research participants of this study: "One woman's story is everyone's story."

Sahra used the silent language of the body (symptoms) and bodily-inscribed story to convey her life experiences. A close reading of her narrative reveals the following language of symptoms:

- Stressed ten times during the detention of the Baha'i leaders during the revolution.
- Distraught when her daughter left for India.
- Depressed when forced to migrate from Iran.
- Hurt and crushed in spirit when her husband's business failed in Japan.
- Sick with worsening diabetes, ulcers and stomach bleeding when her daughter's divorce was finalized.
- Weak and ill when her daughter-in-law died.
- In poor physical and emotional health during the Kobe earthquake.
- Traumatized from the after-effects of the earthquake.
- Lost weight and became sick in Canada when she realized that she would have to depend on her daughter.

Through her life-long experience of pain and suffering, Sahra developed a rich vocabulary of symptoms that she used to tell her story. Only because Sahra is involved in her own act of witnessing—lived reality—does she not tell merely a survival story. Survival in itself, as Frank informs us, is devoid of "any particular responsibility other than continuing to survive" (1995, 66). A relevant question here is this: What is involved in becoming a witness?

First, becoming a witness means taking the responsibility of stating what happened. Sahra considers this to be a life-long calling. Right from the beginning of her story up to the time when she migrates to Canada, Sahra guides the reader to particular events in her life, family and community. The underlying theme conveyed is that of trauma, beginning with childhood and continuing into old age. The issue is not merely of telling but of establishing moral authority. She lets the reader know that she is a witness to pain and suffering because she embodies these experiences, individually and collectively, in the form of a testimony.

Second, we cannot receive this testimony as detached spectators, as witnessing implies a relationship. The kind of hearing required must take into account the presence of the teller, not the content of the story per se but the suffering body of the teller. This impulse calls for "thinking with stories," to use Frank's words, in a way that does not allow one to move on once the story has been heard; the impulse requires one to *live in* the story. In this regard, there is always another story behind the one that has been told. And this story, often untold, is that of systemic and structural oppression, and social injustice brought about by dominant systems of power.

Sahra's story is anchored in a suffering body. To put it another way, it is her body that gives birth to her story. Healing and reconstruction occur when she shares the story with others. This is the first step toward pinpointing the oppression that causes one to suffer in the first place.

Sahra tells her story in Canada in the context of an aging body whose lifelong suffering has not abated but has intensified, as expressed in the metaphor of the house that is not big enough for her shoes. She is saying that if the house does not have space for her shoes—a dispensable item—how will it accommodate her physical, social, cultural and spiritual needs? Sahra is referring to the isolation and confinement that she experiences as a result of being rendered dependent in her old age. Having worked all her life to maintain her freedom and identity as a Baha'i woman, she finds it hard to accept the fact that Canada does not have space for her in her old age. Older people are often denigrated, and the problem is compounded for an immigrant (read: racialized) woman.

Our act of witnessing Sahra's narrative must therefore take into account her present reality as an aging immigrant women, a subject on which Sahra speaks through the language of silence and to which we must now turn. As noted earlier, Sahra does not talk about this part of her life except through one sentence: "I live in a house that does not even have space to keep my shoes."

Aging Immigrant Women
ℬ

It is common knowledge that aging immigrant women have received scant attention in the literature. This is odd, as feminist, ethnic and gerontological studies would gain much from a view anchored in the margins of society. Furthermore, as Lamb (2000) and Dossa (1999) have noted, these various bodies of work would benefit from the inclusion of age. As the foundation story of humankind, age brings into focus elements of "flux, multivocality, change and process" (Lamb 2000, 8).

Substantive erasure of age in these bodies of work may be explained in relation to two factors: categorization of marginal groups into discrete units, and their hierarchical arrangement where age (being old) is relegated to the lowest rung, owing to its low status in society as a dependable service population (Estes 1979). Those who are racialized and gendered (two forms of subordination) fare worse because their social invisibility is compounded. In Canada, for example, older immigrant women (and men) are admitted under the category of dependents as they can only enter the country if they are sponsored by their sons and daughters. This situation translates into a ten-year waiting period for state-based benefits that mainstream older citizens are entitled to by law.

How do we then include age as a social marker in the literature and also in immigration and social service policies? There is no simple answer to this question, only a series of interrogations. First we may note that inclusion of case-study material devoid of epistemology and of the lived reality of people will not take us very far. To reverse the social invisibility of aging immigrant women, we need to keep in mind such questions as the following: How is social knowledge produced, and for whom and for what purpose? (Moore 1996). We also need to recognize that analytical inclusion of age, gender and race (aging women immigrants) brings to light more nuanced perspectives on the working of nation-states. From this point of view we may want to revisit Sahra's life story as a starting point for discussion and reflection on these issues.

It is evident that Sahra's life course has been shaped by the working of the nation-state. In the countries where she lived (Iran, El Salvador, Japan and Canada), state policy determined the circumstances of her life. In Iran, she, her family and her community faced outright persecution, while in the other three countries it was state indifference and apathy that led to her experience of isolation, compounded in Canada by her age. Sahra attributes her depression and state of ill health to this indifference. Non-intervention approaches in the form deprivation of social services and entitlements can be as detrimental as direct but negative intervention such as Othering of racialized minorities.

We must also note that gendering of nation-states has a strong impact on the lives of women, and more so, on minority women. In Sahra's case, in Iran, the martyrdom of largely male members of her family meant that her work in the domestic sphere increased to such an extent that Sahra grew up not knowing what it is like to be a child. Throughout her life, she carried the burden of caring for her family and, by extrapolation, the Baha'i community and the nation-state. Her work for the latter can be appreciated in that women have always played an important role in the formation and reproduction of nations and society. In *Gender and Nation*, for example, Yuval Davis argues that "the discourse on gender and that on nation tend to intersect and be constructed by each other" (1997, 4). On the Middle East front, Abu-Lughod (1998) has noted that nations draw upon images of women to formulate their visions of society and identity. It is important to note that women themselves participate in the debates on citizenship and human rights within particular nation-states and of late globally (Naples and Desai 2002). The Baha'is were central to the formation of the nation-state of Iran. First, they were constructed as renegades who had departed from the state religion of Shi'a Islam. Second, despite their persecution, the Baha'is served Iran well (Kazemzadeh 2000). They provided professional expertise in areas that would otherwise have been bereft of this service (Sahra's husband's work as a travelling teacher is a good example). Note that the Iranian state did not function in isolation. Its policies were governed by Western imperialism (British and American). It is not a coincidence that the banner of the 1978–79 Revolution was anti-imperialism/anti-Westernization. The persecution of the Baha'is was shaped by the Iranian state's articulation with the West. In times when the state felt relatively secure, the persecution of the Baha'is lessened, and with insecurity came increased persecution (Kazemzadeh 2000, Farr 1999). Second, minorities highlight the fault lines of nation-states. An illustrative example is found in *The Dark Side of the Nation*. In this work, Bannerji (2000) argues that the Canadian policy of multiculturalism, initiated by the state supposedly to advance the interests of racialized minorities, in fact serves to contain the tensions between the two founding nations: the French and the British.

Occupying the status of a refugee in El Salvador and Japan and that of a landed immigrant (read: dependent) in Canada, Sahra is in a position to critique these nation-states. Using the silent language of the body—symptoms and bodily-inscribed story—Sahra implicates these societies for rendering her socially invisible, a point that is poignantly brought home by the fact that she does not want her life of pain and suffering to be reduced to nothing. For this reason Sahra acts as a witness to her story with the hope of engaging the readers so that they can live in her story and feel her pain, especially now, in her old age. Sahra calls upon the reader to read her story from within and between spaces of silence and speech.

Notes

1   The participants from the storytelling session were drawn from an ESL class, the parameters of which were defined as "training for integration into Canadian society." Anything beyond this, such as therapeutic storytelling, was dismissed as a waste of scant resources.

2   The funding agency had suggested that Iranian women organize their own storytelling sessions. The Iranian women were reluctant to undertake a depoliticized activity where their voices would not be heard beyond the confines of "an ethnicized community."

3   This woman's story inspired Sahra to participate in the storytelling session vicariously through her daughter.

4   In her work on the elderly Jewish community in California, Myerhoff found that storytelling was the primary means through which members of this community made their presence felt. By and large, this community had been rendered socially invisible.

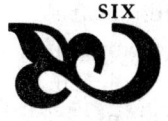

SIX

On Social Suffering:
Fatima's Story

Human suffering has become systemic in our world. Stories of trauma caused by political violence, environmental disasters, civil strife, displacement, and the adverse effects of social policies and practices have become all too common. These occurrences have given rise to a body of literature that has documented the effects of macrosystems on the lived experiences of people (Scheper-Hughes 1992, Das et al. 2001, Das et al. 2000). "Such inquiries, which aim at unveiling the social origins and structural sources of human misery, are particularly crucial for the current historical period, when the dominant voice in the discourse of power persistently and deceitfully insists that responsibility for suffering must be acknowledged by the sufferer himself or herself and thus interprets human suffering in terms of personal stake and individual accountability" (Chuengsatiansup 2001, 31).

The shift from the individual to the social as the cause for human suffering is not easily accomplished as institutional responses mask the workings of the larger system. Institutions isolate and medicalize sufferers to the extent that their lived experiences are appropriated for consumption by global and local audiences. Taking the form of "'infotainment' on the nightly news, images of victims are commercialized; they are taken up into processes of global marketing and business competition" (Kleinman and Kleinman 1997, 1).

Given the above scenario, disciplinary interrogations are at work. Medical anthropologists, in particular, have made a significant contribution towards unmasking the social causes of suffering and pain. Taking a context-specific approach, ethnographers have documented how social suffering and structural violence are mobilized and how these impact on the everyday lives of women and men. Yet, relatively less attention has been given to the political significance of embodied experiences of suffering. This point needs emphasis as human agency is invariably at work, even in the direst situations. The challenge here is to recognize multiple and intricate forms of interventions, keeping in mind that the agency in question is that of people whose social existence has been devalued and silenced by the dominant discourse. Of special importance is the fact that the dominant discourse engages in differential marginalization of people based on such markers as race, class, citizenship and gender. For example, the media construction of racialized women varies from constructs employed by health policy.

Differential workings of power create spaces and cracks between categories and institutional discourses, making it possible for marginalized people to challenge the dominant system and suggest alternative approaches. This chapter addresses this by reading the narrative of one woman: Fatima. Fatima's narrative is of interest to us as it takes us into heart of marginality, where we can observe not only the workings of the dominant discourse but the ways in which it can be challenged.

Profile
ೞ

Fatima immigrated to Canada with her family (husband, daughter and son) in 1991. She was a political refugee but was granted landed immigrant status on the strength of her and her husband's U.S. degrees in economics. The family's attempt to settle down in Montreal was thwarted by overt racism. Resettlement in Vancouver helped Fatima to establish her own import-export business—a protected niche. But this was not for long: Fatima was forced to switch roles and become a full-time caregiver following a car accident in which her daughter incurred brain injury. Fatima felt the need to share her story as she found herself battling on two fronts: coping with discrimination against the disabled, compounded in the case of women of colour, and struggling to have her role as a caregiver/a woman/a mother valorized and legitimated by society.

In this chapter I present Fatima's narrative to provide a broader analysis of her and her daughter's lived experiences. Following an account of Fatima's close encounters with racism, I highlight her points of intervention in a layered landscape that includes everyday life, encounters with the medical system, and the public-private divide that disadvantages women.

Breaking the Silence, Creating a Space for Dialogue

Each time I met with Khadija (an Iranian therapist/counsellor), she told me stories relating to different subjects. In our third meeting, she related what she referred to as "the veil dilemma"—conflicts encountered by women, regardless of whether they chose to wear or discard the veil.[1] On our fourth meeting (March 2001), Khadija informed me that she was in the midst of hearing Fatima's story concerning her daughter's brain injury. Khadija's response to my question on how she establishes contact with Iranian women in crisis was this: "When I find out that a woman is in a difficult situation, I phone her and ask her if she wants to talk." Khadija explained that most women share their stories with her because there are few other opportunities for them to air their concerns. As noted earlier, storytelling does not constitute a mere account of events. It is in fact an active process of reconfiguration of life.

Iranian women wanted to share their stories with Khadija because she was a good listener and not because she was kith and kin. As a counsellor in Iran, she had learned how to prompt women to give expression to their ideas and feelings. But, as I learnt from Fatima, women also wanted to talk to Khadija because they perceived her to be bicultural and bilingual. In other words, she helped women to ground their stories between the spaces of two worlds: home and host.

Like other Iranian women, Khadija could not find work in her area of expertise in Canada. She therefore established a niche that allowed her to validate herself and remember, in her own words, that "women can think and make a significant contribution to society." As a bilingual counsellor, Khadija was invited by mainstream professionals and civil servants to give talks on "Iranian culture." Khadija did not fall into the trap of merely presenting "how-to-do culture"—a stance that has been problematized as it masks the social causes of suffering. Here, the culture of immigrant communities is held responsible for their inability to settle down, when in fact societal and institutional barriers are to blame. While Khadija did not completely abandon the cultural trope—otherwise she would not be invited—she gently implicated the system by telling the stories of women. The women presented these stories in the way of testimonial speaking. Fatima's story is related in this genre.

Fatima told her story to Khadija and myself, separately and together, in eight sessions over a period of eight months. Marmar, her daughter, was present in all the sessions. Although Marmar spoke and participated in the discussions as and when she wanted, she was not the principal participant. Fatima had expressed a desire to tell her story ('tell it all') and we respected her wish. Like Zahra, Fatima also wanted her daughter to hear the full story because Marmar did not remember her experiences following the accident. The meetings took place variously at Fatima's house, Khadija's house and at a restaurant, according to what worked best for everyone. Other than prompting Fatima to elaborate on some aspects, Khadija's role was that of a good listener.

When Khadija first approached Fatima with my inquiry as to whether she was interested in the research project, Fatima jumped at the opportunity. Prior to the storytelling sessions, Fatima submitted the following two paragraphs authored by herself and by her daughter, respectively.

> A therapeutic chance/an opportunity was given to me to review and tell out loud or let it out one of the most devastating experience a woman/mom may experience in her life. Which was: lose a daughter in a long battle of life-threatening situation, and suddenly birth was given to a 19-year-old disabled child in replace. Without having the chance or energy to grieve for the loss of the most precious thing in my life, start another harsh struggle, fighting with all obstacles, limitations and difficulties in life to save her life, and then working for her recovery.

These are my daughter's words to describe her feelings:

The accident on November 22, 1997, changed my life forever. Since I was released from the hospital, I have been depressed and very lonely. Most people have memories of when they were young. However I have forgotten the first twenty years of my life. I can't remember relatives, the places I've been, and the things I've done. This makes me feel like the first twenty years of my life were just a waste. I have lost touch with many of my friends because it was difficult for me to leave my house and in some cases I cannot even remember them. Furthermore, for the past nine months, I have not been able to live like a normal 20-year-old woman. I can no longer live independently and this has caused a great deal of emotional hardship. It devastates me to think that although I am an adult, I cannot take care of myself.

Since the accident, I have become irritable, impulsive, immature and impatient. Often I find myself cursing for no reason, yelling at others and becoming frustrated very easily. My daily life has completely changed for the worst. I need help getting in and out of the shower. I also have trouble going up and down the stairs. For example, before my accident, I used to be able to go dancing with my friends whenever I wanted and for as long as I wanted. However, currently I can no longer dance like I used to and I feel that I am a burden to the people I go out with. Additionally, I've been told that I can't go to a normal school of higher learning or hold a job for two years. When I think about these facts, I begin to wonder if I will ever be normal again.

First reading of the above accounts bring home the devastating impact of a major car accident. Woven into the body of this account is a social script. For Fatima, it is "fighting with all obstacles, limitations and difficulties in life to save her life, and then working for her recovery." Marmar is made to feel that she is a burden on society and she wonders if she will ever be normal again. In a just world, one would expect that one's pain would be lessened by empathy and social support. But this is hardly the case. As Kleinman et al. (1997) and Farmer (2003) have argued, suffering has been rendered into a commodity for consumption by audiences who watch and read about human misery from the comforts of their living rooms. But this is not the end point. There are myriad stories, like those of Fatima and Marmar, that are rendered invisible because they are not considered "worthy" of societal attention. Fatima then takes it upon herself to tell her own story and she does this with vigour and passion. Fatima is also aware that her story will circulate in forums such as the one that Khadija has access to or through print, the medium used by researchers.

Like the Japanese *hibakusha* (bombed) women (Todeschini 2001), Fatima considers it necessary to create a space from which her story will be heard. Such is the silencing of people who are marginalized. Fatima's point of entry is to relate her own experiences of overt racism. In her account, she conveys the injurious effects of racism— an elusive form of suffering. Fatima frames her account in such a way that the reader cannot help but locate what are essentially discrete acts "into a formative relationship with each other, of suggesting a way of thinking them indispensably through each other" (Bannerji 1995, 14). The formative relationship is brought into relief in the reality of everyday life. It is within this realm that trauma and crisis register more deeply. It is also within this space that acts of resistance take place. This context paves the way for Fatima to relate her account of societal response to her daughter's brain injury.

✷ Telling Her Story of Border Crossing

Fatima came to Canada with the expectation that she and her family (husband, 15-year-old daughter and 11-year-old son) would be well received. Fatima believed that she had the right credentials: she and her husband were political refugees, they both had master's degrees in economics from United States, and they were young. From the point of view of the Canadian state, they were desirable immigrants who would hit the ground running. Fatima and her husband wanted no less. They were keen to settle down quickly and for this reason they decided to live in Montreal: "We were told that it is easier to get jobs here and this is the reason why we went to Montreal." Fatima encountered a world different from the one she had envisioned.

We moved to Montreal and spent whatever we had saved in Iran in three years. We spend around $125,000. My husband [Mohammed] with his economic background took on a job of a door-to-door salesperson. Even though he was a shy person. There was no other way to live. All these were tortures for him. In our culture there was no such thing as commission job. He could not change his personality but he went through a lot of torture. We received no help from the Iranian community. We never found a reliable job in Montreal.

Note that Fatima first talks about her husband before relating her own experiences. This is because women's subordinate status makes it necessary for them to create their own spaces and establish moral authority before they speak. By highlighting her husband's suffering ("tortures"), Fatima positions herself to tell her tale from the socially valorized role of a wife. Fatima then talks about her distress in not being able to find work in her area of expertise. She intertwines her personal experiences with a collective story of mistreatment of her people in Canada.

The job that I had found in Montreal was at a very low level. I did not have Canadian experience. I was not accepted/trusted for any jobs. We felt that people had preconceptions about us as being Iranian. People had stereotypes about us, and that is how we would get treated. Fear of financial insecurity affected my relationship with my husband and children. We could not provide a healthy environment for our children.

He would go to twenty places each day looking for a job. When I looked for a job, I would not say that I have a master's degree in economics from the United States. I thought to myself this degree was working against me. When I came here, I registered in a computerized accounting programme, and the school asked me for a resume. I did not write that I have a degree.

In Montreal with the deposit in our bank account, we could not even lease a car. We need someone to come and co-sign for us, someone that has lived there. Even if we wanted to rent a place we needed a co-signer, someone that has a job, and knows us. *Silent, she shakes her head, and then continues.*

Immigrant women's ties to the marketplace are tenuous and ambiguous. They are largely sought for work in the lower echelons of the labour force and are dispensed with once these positions are eliminated. The ambiguity arises from the fact that the labour of these women is desirable but remains unacknowledged. Acknowledging immigrant women's contributions would mean improving their working conditions, a situation that a profit-based system avoids at all costs. The system in fact deploys the socially constructed categories of race and gender to secure a cheap source of labour. Capitalistic systems are gendered and raced. These observations reveal that Fatima's entry at the lower rungs of the labour force is not coincidental. It is structural, and this aspect prompts Fatima to hide her qualifications, despite the fact that they were acquired in a place (U.S.) where her credentials would not be an issue. A low-end position does not spare Fatima from racism that translates into violence of her self/her body.

> They could not accept me between themselves. I would think that I'm boring. I had my own value system. I tried very hard to be accepted. I wasted my time. I even got more humiliated—that made me very angry. I needed to be accepted by them. If I attended a party, no one would even talk to me or even look at me. They gave me the feeling of, "I am really disgusted, why you want to get into our group, get out." I could not be myself.

Das and Kleinman suggest that "the experience of subjugation may itself, when owned and worked upon, become the source of claiming a subject position" (cf. Butler 2001, 6). But in reality, such positions are not claimed with facility and when they do exist, they need to be teased out. This process is revealed in two contexts in the narrative.

First is the crossing of boundaries from the personal to the political. The issue of boundary crossing concerning the moment when an individual gains political consciousness has been subject to debate. One body of work suggests that this form of consciousness requires the availability of the right set of circumstances such as grass-root level movements, a particular crisis, or a critical exposure to the workings of the dominant system (Fiona 2001, Todeschini 2001). A second body of work foregrounds the premise that the personal is political regardless of circumstances except that this awareness is latent and may be brought to light through such mediums as stories (Scheper-Hughes 1992).

The moment Fatima stated that she had to hide her qualifications, she entered the political arena. She is suggesting that there must be something amiss in a society that compels people to hide their real qualifications. In making this statement, Fatima reinforced insights from the literature produced by women of colour and transnational feminists, indicating that women of colour are looked upon as a source of cheap labour that can be dispensed with according to the needs of the market (Naples and Desai 2002). In such a situation, as Bannerji (1995) has argued, the bodies of women of colour in white collar jobs are an anomaly.

Fatima crosses yet another boundary: from speech to the silent language of the body. *"Silent, she shakes her head, and then continues."* When the body speaks, it conveys a politically charged message (Frank 1995). Fatima conveys the message that she has no words to describe the suffering and the pain caused by social exclusion and racism—the soft knife of politics. Farmer (2003) and Bannerji (1995) have respectively noted that the effects of racism are injurious. The wounds go deep and impact on one's sense of well-being and identity as a person. But there is no closure. People who fight back must also be listened to, because they bring to light the elements of a just world. A first and important step in this direction is to recognize their subjectivity.

The second context is transnational. Being aware of the colonial discourse on the veil/*hejab* which Others Muslim women (Alvi et al. 2003), Fatima takes the reader to her country of birth. She notes that even if she wore the *hejab* in Iran as compelled by the state, she did not lose her identity or dignity. Her work as an economist was recognized and valued. Nevertheless, she does not romanticize her country of birth. She admits that in Iran she was suspected of being a U.S. spy, and that she was pressurized to stay at home by the government's ideological stance that "a woman belongs to the house." These were the two reasons why Fatima left Iran. Yet, for Fatima, these experiences pale in comparison with what she lived through in her adopted country. "I am pushed to lose my identity." "At work," she continued, "they would often talk about immigrant frauds. What should I say ... it is better I go"—that is, she does not want to talk any more. Silence, once again, implicates the system.

Fatima's experiences in the Canadian labour force form part of a structural moment. Long before Fatima stepped into the office, her low-paid work (downward mobility), along with the attitudes and behaviour of her co-workers, were determined by the racialized and gendered Canadian immigration policy (Thobani 1999, Gupta 1996). The policy stipulates that, by and large, women are desirable immigrants only because they are the source of cheap labour that can fill positions that no one else wants to occupy. Of late, immigrant women constitute a pool of volunteers in the downsized social service sector. The fact that Fatima was granted landed immigrant status based on her (also her husband's) U.S. qualifications is of no consequence. Once in the country, the racialized and gendered system channelled her into entry-level work, just as it did Nadia. During a low financial period in their lives, Fatima and her husband applied for welfare.

> They [social service staff] would not let us in. We would often hear, "if you want to leave it [application], but it is going to end up in the garbage." Often in the hallways, on my way from one office to the other, I felt humiliated and cried. I wanted to work for free for three months. My offer was not accepted even on humanitarian basis. It was not their fault because the economic system here does not give them this choice. According to my experience, society does not accept/respect new immigrants. For example, I remember as a new immigrant when I stepped in the coffee room at the office I used to work, they would stop their conversation.

The feminist project in anthropology has been informed by three phases: to make women visible as historical, social, economic and political actors; to foreground gender as a central analytical category;

and to recognize the tightly woven link between gender and social institutions (De Groot 1996). What is of interest in Fatima's account is her point of intervention in this project. Through the sheer act of narration of such events as the incident in the hallway and her encounters in the coffee room, Fatima establishes her position as a political actor. Her implication of the system (society's belittling of immigrant women) does not focus merely on individuals ("it was not their fault"). She concentrates on institutional power and as such her message is a political one that can be placed on a par with critical ethnography. Here the emphasis is on dialogue where "anthropological knowledge may be seen as something produced in human interaction, not merely 'extracted' from native informants who are unaware of the hidden agendas coming from the outsider" (Scheper-Hughes 1992, 25). The issue here is that this approach should not be the exclusive preserve of anthropologists. Research participants may initiate dialogue that evokes the presence of a listening community. Fatima initiates this process through the narrative act where the emphasis is not only on what she says but on how she frames her account. Fatima withdraws and shares information according to her own political project, an important component of which is her gendered identity as a mother and a professional woman.

Unable to stand the humiliation and the pain that Fatima and her husband were subject to in Montreal, the couple moved to Vancouver to make a fresh start. Fatima glossed over this part of her life. She explained that she worked for a firm for three years and then started her own export-import business. This enclave sheltered her from the pain and the humiliation that she experienced in Montreal. She hoped to bury this part of her life, but not for long. Her daughter's accident made it necessary for her to talk about these experiences, if for no other reason than to claim another subject position from which she could speak: that of a caregiver. Fatima found herself carrying the societal burden of care and this social load compelled her to tell her story. Recall her words: "A therapeutic chance/an opportunity was given to me to review and tell out loud or let it out one of the most devastating experience a women/mom may experience in her life."

Bearing the Societal Burden of Care
ಏಿ

As a mom, how I feel about a disabled child. As a mother to protect my child I support her, help her to develop ability and skill to live in the society and protect herself against discrimination that exist against her, not just the right to work or equal opportunity. To protect her from psychological damage. Society here as soon as they see a disabled person, they think of him/her as a lesser person (I mean majority) since there are few who accept and see it any other way of being in this world not just be as someone incapable. However, in public, people don't respect your physical limitation.

These are Fatima's first words on her role as a mother and a caregiver. Unlike people with stories of multiple sclerosis (Monks and Frankenberg 1995), Fatima does not focus exclusively on the adjustment that she and her daughter have to make. For Fatima, the issue concerns societal response to her daughter's brain injury. For Marmar, living in a different body translates into societal rejection of her as a person. She is perceived as a burden, a situation that she internalizes.

Including but also moving beyond the adjustment script takes Fatima into the heart of what disability scholar Oliver (1996) refers to as "disability as social oppression." This form of oppression is multi-dimensional: social, economic, cultural and psychological. Fatima was compelled to deal with this complex scenario. At one level, she took on the position of a full-time caregiver because Marmar had to start from scratch. Fatima explained that she had to teach her daughter such things as "how to walk" and "how to hold a fork." Rather than receiving any societal support or recognition for her work, Fatima found herself waging a battle against denigration of disabled people, compounded for racialized minorities and women (Asce and Fine 1988, Dossa 2000). This is what Fatima has to say:

When I go to Marmar to a concert, mall, or cinema, even in college people don't care about her physical disability. They brush her off. Here people just care about their own business. In a sense selfish, they are self-centred. They don't want to bother to spare any minute of their life for a lesser person (disabled). When she walks with a cane, no one is considerate, to let her go first or slow down so that they don't hit her. Or let her get into the elevator first, or wait a minute for her to get in.

Societal oppression of the disabled does not exclude family members. Referring to Marmar's visit to her cousins in United States, Fatima observed,

They would walk ahead in the restaurant, and for Marmar she could not walk fast. This brought her a bad feeling. Feeling such as being leftover, not wanted, a burden. "I wish I had not gone" is what Marmar said. We are talking about a young adult who is full of life, full of sense of humour and also very intelligent whenever her mental difficulties do not come out as an obstacle.

Medical anthropologists have brought to our attention the multi-faceted dimensions of what appears to be existential human suffering (Kleinman et el. 1997, Das et al. 2001). First is the corporeal-bodily reality that in disability literature is referred to as impairment (Corker and French 1999). Second is the focus on social conditions such as political conflict, forced migration, and the adverse impact of state policies and practices on communities and individuals. These two levels of suffering are intensified by insensitive institutional and bureaucratic responses that isolate sufferers and subject them to medicalization.

The third dimension of suffering involves the exercise of human agency, which serves a twofold purpose. First, it prevents total appropriation of suffering by the larger and increasingly global systems of power. As Kleinman and Kleinman have noted: "This globalization of suffering is one of the most troubling signs of the cultural transformation of the current era: troubling because experience is being used as a commodity, and through this cultural representation of suffering, experience is being remade, thinned out and distorted" (1997, 2). Second, human agency points to alternative ways that have the potential to effect social change. Note that these ways are not confined to a discrete sphere but exist alongside or in the midst of dominant systems.

A close reading of Fatima's narrative text reveals all the above dimensions. To begin with, Fatima and her daughter highlight the issue of impairment. For Fatima, this means becoming a full-time caregiver. For Marmar, impairment is conveyed in her own words: difficulties in climbing stairs instead of dancing.

Social factors are not easily implicated in a car accident because individuals are held responsible for this occurrence. If we were to engage in what Farmer (2003) refers to as "geographically broad and historically deep analysis," we would be able to establish a correlation between accident-based injuries/death and the social order (read: profit-drive market system). In essence, car accidents are a result of high volume of automobile traffic that has left little room for pedestrians, cyclists and also public transport. Automobile manufacture, a profit-making industry, epitomizes the capitalistic system. This system's negative impact on the environment and the lives of people is masked by a host of supporting institutions. Given this dense scenario, Fatima does not focus on the cause of the accident. She invests her energy in highlighting societal response to her daughter's brain injury. Through her account of particular incidents in her and her daughter's everyday life (concert, elevator, restaurant), she brings home the social cause of suffering.

Focus on everyday reality is important as it is in this realm that pain and suffering register more poignantly; it is also within this space that social interactions take place and where our bodies' multi-faceted reality is shaped. Equally important is the fact that everyday life is not detached from the larger hegemonic systems that operate in a way so as to make us believe that this reality is a commonsense and taken-for-granted aspect of life. Fatima grounds her experiences in this realm but also expands them to include a transnational dimension. She takes the reader to her home country in Iran "to heal Marmar's wounds." What Fatima and her daughter lived through was day-to-day discrimination experienced on the basis of intersecting inequalities of gender and race and disability. While Fatima bases her narrative on disability, issues of gender and race (Iranian women) are also in the forefront.

The way they treat her, the way they approach her, the way they care about her, the impact all this kind of support is that she would feel as accepted, respected and loved as much, if not even more as if she did not have this disability. I took her to Iran to save her heart. To repair her soul because here [in Canada] she was not feeling very much loved, or accepted. She lacked emotional nourishment. The worst of all, she lost all her friends after the accident. She became lonely and all of them disappeared, then she had her major struggle. She was trying so hard to bring back her friends, which did not happen. She was so disappointed she felt as no one loves her, no one wants to be around her because she is disabled.

But in Iran she was in middle of the crowd, and one of them. One among others, one of them like any others or in another word, to be accepted. A mother understands things that others can't. I could understand her needs. To nurture her spirit and to repair her broken heart, give her a chance to feel good again even with all her disabilities and difficulties. You are as much, if not more, loved and respected, cared as before this incident.

In *Disability and Culture,* Whyte and Ingstad (1995) put forward the method of cultural juxtaposition that enables anthropologists to draw insights from other societies and apply them to problems in their own societies. This anthropological tradition is subject to debate on two grounds. First, there is the danger that the West—the dominant and home territory of anthropologists—would be the reference point for comparison; second, this tradition promotes a divide between the West and the Rest. The latter is considered to have a subordinate status even within the realm of international organizations. Drawing upon her experiential knowledge as a caregiver and as a person who has lived in both the worlds, Fatima engages with this debate.

Fatima's trip to Iran was prompted by a lack in her country of re-settlement. This lack relates to the issue of personhood "seen as being not simply human but human in a way that is valued and meaningful" (Ibid., 10). Why is it the case that in the Western world disability is equated with social oppression? This question does not imply that persons with disabilities are free of oppression in other parts of the world. What is required is a context-specific framework within which to study disability in any society. Taking a socio-historical perspective, Striker contends that the status of the disabled people in the Western world is best explained in relation to a centralist state. The state has appropriated the lives of disabled persons in a way that renders them dependent and needy. "Thus disability in Europe and North America exists within—and is created by—a framework of state, legal, economic and biomedical institutions. Concepts of personhood, identity, and value, while not reducible to institutions, are nevertheless shaped by them" (cf. Whyte and Ingstad, 10).

Fatima does not comment on the status of the disabled in Iran. To do so would have diluted her context-specific script involving everyday life situations. She focuses on particular but crucial spaces such as that of being in a crowd or among a group of people. Here Marmar is not treated as a lesser person because of her disability. To reiterate Fatima's words, "But in Iran she was in middle of the crowd, and one of them. One among others, one of them like any other or in another word to be accepted." Acceptance in a group/crowd that otherwise did not know Marmar as an individual gave her the assurance that her life is worth living and that she was not a burden on society. In short, Marmar was not marked as negatively different because of her disability.

Fatima established a "link" between Iran and Canada by providing a context as to what prompted her to visit Iran.

> My feeling about taking her to Iran for psychological treatment became a sure idea when my sister [Forouzan] from Iran came to support and help me and Marmar. My sister's three months of therapeutic services that she provided was like a breakthrough point in Marmar's recovery.

Forouzan's visit to Canada was made possible by the support that she received from her family in Iran. The family (natal and marital) collected funds for her trip and they took care of her children while she was away. Forouzan also made a personal sacrifice as she took an unpaid leave of absence from her teaching job. Through the care and emotional support that she provided to Marmar, Fatima came to know what she lacked in Canada.

Whyte and Ingstad (1995) offer useful comparative insights on attitudinal differences towards disabled persons. They argue that North American society has little to offer to disabled persons as it medicalizes and individualizes their lives—approaches that depoliticize struggles for justice and equality. The opposite situation prevails in the South. There, disabled persons are not subject to essentialized identities ("wheelchair bound" as opposed to "wheelchair user") owing to minimal institutional control. Ironically, the latter translates into minimal state-based services, leaving the family to take care of disabled members. Fatima does not reject the institutional services that Marmar needs for her recovery: physiotherapy, occupational therapy, speech therapy and psychological counselling. Her activism is based on the conviction that the disabled in the West do not receive emotional support, thus reducing their chances to socially interact and ultimately compromising their sense of who they are as people.

> In this [Western] culture, there is less emotional support. This society is run by laws [read: institutionalization]. But in Iranian culture, people's support is not generated by law and if they see a disabled person they volunteer to help. They automatically give priority to disabled person. In the eighteen months after Marmar's accident, I realized the need to take her back to Iran for emotional support.

> I want to talk about Iran. In Iran everybody first sympathize with a handicap person. There you can have a normal life. Emotionally less under pressure. Here a person is separated from society, and doesn't feel as one with other members of society. One of the biggest pains of a disabled person is that his/her life is separated from everyone else, separated from her old environment. In her new environment she is lonely with no love. This is a major suffering. In Iran, even though people might look at her with pity, nobody behaves around her in a way so that she would feel sorry for herself. She had had the feeling of acceptance, the same amount of love she still would get from people surrounding her the same as before her disabilities.

In taking issue with institutional services that separate the individual from society, Fatima enters into the heart of one of the main concerns expressed in the literature on social suffering. This body of work is based on the premise that institutions and social conditions must be implicated in all forms of human suffering. Even if human misery cannot directly be linked to societal factors, it is intensified by societal insensitivity and further marginalization of the sufferers.

❧ Battling on Two Fronts

Fatima related that she had to wage a battle on two fronts. First there was her daughter, Marmar. Fatima felt her pain very deeply. She could not bear to see the agony that Marmar was going through as she struggled to build her life from scratch. Such activities as walking, eating, taking a bath and dressing were new to her. Marmar's attempts to relearn what she had learned over nineteen years of her life were frustrated by the obstacles that society placed before her. Fatima related that even going to the doctor was a struggle because she had to help Marmar get dressed and drive her to his office. Yet, every time they went (a couple of times a month), the doctor made them wait for as long as forty-five minutes. It was hard for Marmar to sit this long. Once they were late by fifteen minutes and the doctor shouted at them and said that they were wasting his precious time. It was the same doctor who advised Fatima to "forget" about Marmar as, in his words, "The accident happened and there is nothing more you can do." Fatima gave other examples of insensitivity, such as how Marmar was drugged to numb her pain when all that she needed was a massage from a nurse; how the nurses would shout at her when she did not want to take a shower; how they would take their time to change her position on the bed to prevent sores and so on.

The dehumanized care that Marmar received during her eighteen-month stay at the hospital was not remedied by the outside world.[2] Marmar's experiences are captured in statements cited at the beginning of this chapter. When Fatima realized that society was shunning its responsibility towards the disabled, she took the societal burden onto her own shoulders. This made her fight a second battle: that of ensuring that society recognize her role as a caregiver.

> I wish that the society or government agencies recognize and appreciate the twenty-four hours of services that I was providing.

As the result of me losing my job, a household of two incomes suffered financially and that created lots of problems. Something that I did not need at that time. That job of taking care of a brain-injured young adult is very painful and difficult. If you add to all these difficulties, financial difficulties, you can imagine how bad the situation can get. I wish that government would compensate at least minimum wage for eight hours a day. A service that was essential for Marmar's recovery. If I did not do what I did, she would have never recovered as much, and she would be left as a disabled who would need twenty-four hours of intensive care. What I am trying to say is that they should recognize the benefit of these services provided with love to a fellow citizen and society. At least compensate a portion of it for the sake of a healthy society.

Aside from dealing with the issue of recognition, Fatima was belittled and considered "stupid" for not getting on with her life. "Can you not understand that brain-injured people's recovery lasts a lifetime? How can you not get on with your own life?" This is the message that Fatima heard from medical specialists. Consider the following critical incidents.

First, Fatima related, her psychiatrist, who was helping her cope with stress and depression, "threw me out of her office. She said that if I was not willing to put my daughter in a group home, there is nothing more she can do for me." Second, the psychiatrist's views were reinforced by family members: her husband and brother-in-law urged her to get on with her life. They told her that it was not her fault that the accident happened. Fatima explained that her husband did not "see" how much care she was putting into Marmar's recovery. She attributes the invisibility of her work to the fact that "the government does not pay for the full-time work that I put into my daughter's care." Fatima explained that if she were to put her daughter into a group home, it would cost the government a lot of money. Fatima felt that even a minimum wage would enhance her status as a caregiver.

To make her case, Fatima highlighted the multi-faceted nature of caregiving. She states that a good caregiver first has to become a student and learn about the person that she is caring for. In her case, she had to learn whatever she could about brain injury, but this was not sufficient. She also had to learn about Marmar as a whole person and not as an individual splintered by her disability. This meant relating to Marmar emotionally but also being cognizant of details concerning her body: sore points, balance, coordination and so on. Added to this enormous task were the societal prejudices and discrimination that Fatima had to confront and whose elimination she had to work towards. As Wendell has expressed it: "[D]isability is socially constructed through the failure or unwillingness to create ability among people who do not fit the physical and mental profile of 'paradigm' citizens. Failure of social support for people with disabilities results in inadequate rehabilitation ... and many other disabling situations that hurt people with disabilities and exclude them from participation in major aspects of life in their societies" (1996, 40).

Disability scholars have argued that disabled people are treated as lesser beings who do not count and whose lives can be dispensed with through such means as abortion of "defected" fetuses, incarceration and gross disregard for their quality of life (Wendell 1996, Oliver 1996). The struggles of disabled persons then begin at the level of basic rights and entitlements that able-bodied people take as given: accessibility, employment, schooling, parenting, sexuality, health and others. Further, disabled people are labelled as Other and subjected to stigma at multiple levels, compounded in the case of racialized women and other socially disadvantaged minorities. It is these multi-faceted concerns that prompted Fatima to become a full-time caregiver.

Caregiving is not confined to task-oriented work, as common wisdom has it. While this work is crucial (Fatima says that her daughter would have been in a wheelchair if she had not worked towards her recovery), there are other dimensions that are equally daunting and challenging. These dimensions concern overcoming the long-standing Cartesian dichotomy (bed-body work versus social relations) and dealing with societal barriers where disability is nothing less than oppression. For Fatima, caregiving is a mission that she had to undertake; no one around her understood Marmar's needs as a whole person and not a splintered human being. But in the process, Fatima herself was denigrated.

It is a fact that my husband, or even my husband's family, looked at me as an unemployed person. I have lost my self-respect as a professional working woman with a good salary. For three and a half years in the pain of being a nobody, and the feelings that you are only worthy and valued when you bring money home. And I was not able to work anymore because of Marmar; because Marmar's sickness was a mental sickness and I had to always educate myself about her condition and I wanted to be involved in all the therapy sessions so that I would be more informed on what has happened to Marmar and to learn the treatments. And thirdly to be able to follow the practices at home so that I would be more beneficial to her.

And I was the only person that was filling Marmar's loneliness, there was no one else. Her friends were gone as well, and had left her alone. I was her friend, her therapist, massage therapist, her teacher, that was a very hard job, and I had to teach myself on how to work with Marmar. This meant that I was a full-time student so that I could learn so that I could treat Marmar better. A lot of time I had to observe Marmar carefully to find a solution for her problem. I had to create a chart to record all her activities and pain so that I would be able to understand where her pain was coming from.

If the government could provide minimum wage for all these services that I am giving as a mother this would lessen the pressures that have been building up, and maybe I would not be forced to break under all these pressures, and feel the need to see a therapist, and take prescription drugs for my own health.

The question that Fatima raises in her account is this: Why does society not reward a person who takes on multiple roles (teacher, massage therapist, therapist, friend) to take care of another person (in her words, "service from one human being to another")? Aside from the issue of reward, we may state that the person is actually punished. Fatima stated that she lost her social status and her health was jeopardized because society took no notice of her full-time work with Marmar. For a response to the above question, we may turn to the literature.

Caregiving evokes the lesser and more discrete world of home that is run and managed by women. This is a contrived setup put into place by the state, which is interested in securing the unpaid labour of women within a space that remains socially invisible. Furthermore, the state has taken full advantage of the gendered ideology that women by nature are caring, loving, gentle and sacrificial beings. Feminist intervention into this political economy script has been vigorous. In her work on family caregiving, Anne Opie (1992) suggests that we pay close attention to the way in which what are presented as separate spheres are in fact closely intertwined. This is contrary to the stance taken by the state. Opie argues that the private sphere of home is indeed shaped by social, economic and political contexts. To effect any kind of change, we need to implicate these contexts. Devaluation of persons providing care translates into devaluation of persons receiving care, and thus it is necessary for us, argues Opie, to deconstruct this conflation. The task of making visible the work of the caregivers is rendered more difficult in the wake of downsizing and privatization of social service programmes, a development that has made the state focus on "community care" that assumes the availability of unpaid female caregivers. The solution proposed by Opie is to question the private and the public divide that the state uses to its benefit—a task that Fatima undertakes based on her experiential knowledge on caregiving. In her own words,

> From the first day, I did not leave this kid alone as part of being a mother. But it has to be recognized that if it was not for my care this kid would have suffered from another brain injury and not recover as much. The government and society should pay the huge cost of recovery. This did not occur because I was there to take care of her with passion. As a women and a mother, I suffered in many ways. It all returns to that the government does not recognize and respect biological and natural rights of a free caregiver, who is a mother. It would cost the government more in the end, if I leave this service!

In this passage, Fatima made a strong case to have her services as a caregiver recognized by the state and by the society. She framed her argument in the language that the state would understand: cost effectiveness. At the same time, she highlighted the enormous cost that she has to bear: "I suffered in many ways." She continues,

> The whole time I have to struggle with my husband, and myself so that I don't lose my self-esteem because I am always under attack. Because of financial pressures my spouse wanted me to return back to work, and it was me that would not leave this kid alone to return to work even though the whole family was in need of money. If society recognized the value of my services, my family who is also a part of society will also respect my work as well.

Of interest is the fact that the blurring of the boundaries between the public and the private takes place on the shifting grounds of identity. Fatima refers to herself as a woman, a mother and a caregiver. The convergence but also disjuncture of these roles—a woman is not invariably a caregiver and, for Fatima, this was especially the case as before the accident she identified herself as a professional woman—makes a powerful script of sacrifice but also highlights the politics of care as revealed in the following passage: "I have a serious claim as a women and as a mother. If I was respected for the care I provide with love, my husband would also understand and appreciate what I am doing." The message conveyed is that she is still a working woman, but on the home front. This intervention—her own take and understanding of the situation—subverts the public/private divide. It is within this deconstructed space that Fatima tells her story and in the process identifies a niche for remaking a world that is otherwise filled with suffering and pain.

Concluding Note

&

We began this chapter with the observation that social suffering is multi-faceted. In particular we noticed that social suffering can either be appropriated or else rendered invisible by the dominant system. Social suffering is also not easy to document in a world where it is taken as a common occurrence that takes place out there in another part of the world. Our role in this respect is to consume images of suffering that the media presents to us in a framework that absolves us from any responsibility both as observers and as participants in a system that isolates sufferers. We have also observed that this political economy script is not complete. People who are subjected to pain and suffering do not maintain silence. They feel the need to tell their stories, often in the form of testimonial speaking.

An intriguing aspect of stories is that they do not exist within a discrete sphere of what the dominant system refers to as "their culture and therefore their stories." In other words, the dominant group would like to hear stories that do not implicate it in any way. As noted in the example of the refugee hearing process, the stories that are validated are those that portray the West as a saviour of people from the Third World. The latter is portrayed as uncivilized where chaos and violence are the order of the day. Given this scenario, stories of marginalized people act as points of intervention into the hegemonic system. While such stories hold the system accountable for their plight, they go beyond this level to include alternative discourses and strategies. Such is the context in which Fatima tells her story.

Through the deployment of narrative strategies—the how, what and when of storytelling—Fatima first claimed a subject position from which she can speak with authority. Fatima's awareness of the working of the system based on the intersections of inequality of such markers as race, gender and disability came during the early period of her settlement. Her exclusion and marginalization was total as it not only kept her away from the work that she is qualified to do but affected her sense of identity and well-being. Fatima's implication of the racialized system is intriguing. She uses the colonial narrative of the veil (read: oppression of Muslim women by Islam) to bring into relief an ironic situation: "Even when I wore the veil, I did not lose my identity. I was valued for my work. Here in Canada I cannot be myself. You are pushed to lose your identity." The message conveyed is to the effect that it is the structural location of immigrant women—lack of opportunities for work and full development of their capacities—that determines their life chances. In her example of the veil and its linkage with women's work, Fatima reverses the hierarchy where the West presents itself as superior and democratic.

Note that Fatima shares her story of re-settlement to lay the groundwork for telling yet another story from the margins of the margins. This second story's marginal status arises from the fact that the issue of disability has not been incorporated into the race/gender/ class paradigm. Yet, disability contains intricate layers. The starting point is the existential form of suffering and pain (impairment), intensified by institutional response. It is important to understand how this response is mobilized within particular contexts and in terms of specific discourses. Fatima's narrative provides insights on these aspects. Through her depiction of everyday life situations, we come to know how Marmar's struggle for recovery is made worse by societal indifference and rejection of her racialized, gendered and disabled body. Everyday life is layered, as it is at this level that pain and suffering are brought into greater relief. Within the space of everyday life, resistance, especially in scattered forms, is exercised.

In the context of everyday life, and between the spaces of the private and the public, Fatima wages her battles: to take care of her brain-injured daughter in a way that goes well beyond what is referred to as bed-and-body work (the physical aspects of recovery). Fatima gives equal and special emphasis to nurturing "Marmar's soul," to use her words. It is for this reason that she takes her daughter to Iran. Reversing the anthropological tradition of cultural juxtaposition, Fatima brings to the fore particular spaces to provide an example of healing of the soul. She uses this example to critique the Western approach that separates the individual from society—a practice that Fatima considers to be injurious to one's well-being. We learn that this form of separation is politically motivated as it absolves society from bearing any responsibility. Canadian society and, more broadly, the West pushes disabled people into the private sphere where they are rendered socially invisible. Fatima ensures that this private space is made public by relating particular incidents that impact on Marmar's recovery and sense of well-being.

Fatima also takes on the project of making visible women's work in the private sphere. She presents a powerful script of how her sense of well-being, dignity and self-worth are negatively affected because society does not validate her full-time work as a teacher, a therapist, a woman, a mother and a caregiver. Her suggestion that the government should compensate her for this work subverts the public-private divide. She effectively conveys the message that her work in the private sphere should be a societal concern. In light of the fact that neither institutional nor civic society will take responsibility for Marmar, Fatima shouldered the societal burden of care but not without implicating the system and suggesting alternative discourse that kept alive the idea that the private sphere is an integral part of the public sphere.

Note that the speaker is a racialized woman who is effectively given the societal message "You can speak and take action if you like but do not move into our territory. Whatever you do must be confined to your own 'community' and 'culture.'" Referred to as the script of containment of minorities to spaces and places that do not shake the world of the dominant majority, this practice has worked well because the state can continue with its business without having to recognize substantive citizenship rights of this group (Dossa 1999, 2000).

The public-private divide contains other dichotomies such as disability and impairment, emotion and reason, law and sociality, and the West and its Other. Fatima's narrative takes on special meaning because she speaks from between these divided spaces. It is from these spaces that Fatima seeks recognition for herself and her daughter for who they are: whole human beings and not splintered subjects.

Notes

1   It must be noted that these conflicts arise from external factors. A Muslim woman is "judged" regardless of whether she is veiled or unveiled. A veiled woman is looked down upon as someone who refuses to "integrate" into Canadian society and also as someone who is tradition-bound (read: oppressed). An unveiled woman may also be frowned upon as someone who has become "too Westernized." This dilemma is highlighted in the video documentary *The Green Light*.

2   Fatima stated that the only time Marmar received "good care" was when she was in the Intensive Care Unit. Once she moved to the regular ward, Marmar received the kind of care that is commonly referred to as "bed-and-body" work. Here the emphasis is on personal hygiene. Fatima then felt it necessary to stay with Marmar every day until late at night. She wants society to recognize her work: "If society as a whole put value on my work, my family who is part of society will also respect my work." In her words, she could then give her daughter the kind of holistic care that a human being is entitled to.

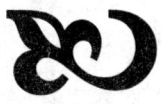

Conclusion:
Re-imagining Mental Health and Well-being

Medical anthropologists have been at the forefront in addressing the disjunction between biomedicine and official discourses on health, and "storied expressions" (embodied knowledge) by laypeople. Lock and Kaufert (1998), Kleinman et al. (1997) and Scheper-Hughes (1992), among others, argue that laywomen and -men adopt multiple positions to challenge and transform medicalized discourses on health. Lock and Kaufert make the point that people on the margins do not act within discrete spheres that would isolate them further. Rather, their point of intervention includes selectively adopting and/ or resisting dominant models. This is a strategic move as it illustrates people's subjectivity. Through stories and narratives we can observe this complex form of resistance and reconfiguration.

Storytelling has a wide scope. It includes the language of silence, it subverts the dominant Cartesian dichotomy (subject/object, public/private), and it evokes responses from a listening community. These are the contexts discussed in this book—contexts that allow us to see how the post-revolution cohort of Iranian women express and re-imagine issues of mental health and well-being. As each woman speaks, she implicates the system. This point needs emphasis, as marginalized communities are often considered to work within the confines of their own traditions and cultures. Their critique of the larger system is barely acknowledged. As well as bringing to light their suffering and experiences of mental ill health, the women in this study identify alternative pathways using the only avenue that is open to them, and that is storytelling. Mental health, broadly defined as social suffering, and its narrative reconstitution on the plane of displacement form the subject matter of this chapter.

Mental Health and Suffering

❧

It has long been established that mental health is not confined to the medical realm but includes institutional practices and discourses as well as public spaces such as the workplace and everyday life. Yet, this established co-relation between mental health and social factors has not been put into practice; neither has it been theorized from the point of view of sufferers. On-the-ground treatment of people diagnosed as "depressed" is informed by biomedicine stipulating that mental health is primarily an issue of genetics and chemical imbalance. The parameters of the Diagnostic and Statistical Manual IV—the fountainhead of modern psychiatry—considers social precursors as secondary. Das and Kleinman (2001) observe that one's already compromised mental health or trauma can be further jeopardized by societal insensitivity and bureaucratic (read: dehumanized) procedures. Having had the benefit of cross-cultural studies, medical anthropologists have made a case for a paradigm shift from the Cartesian dichotomy, which governs our understanding and treatment of mental health, to a more holistic and politically informed approach. However, this broader understanding of mental health has not taken root. The present system with its demarcated spheres, such as the individual and the society, the private and the public, and the body and the mind, masks structural factors that have an impact on people's health and well-being. Furthermore, the current trend towards downsizing and privatization of health care has frustrated the implementation of innovative and more humane models of care.

The multicultural makeup of Canadian society highlights the need to include issues of gender, race, class and other markers of difference in mental health delivery. Research in this area has primarily taken the Band-Aid approach as opposed to implicating the institutional structures. Medical schools and biomedical practice have yet to address the issue of difference, systematically and critically. In metropolis Vancouver, the field site of this study, there are no mental health or community organizations that substantively address the issue of difference. Critical scholarship suggests that it is best to look at the issue of difference in terms of intersecting inequalities, as people's identities are multiple and cannot be contained within one marker such as gender but not ethnicity, or class but not race (Moore 1995, Bannerji 2000, Jiwani 2001, Dyck 1995).

Service organizations have addressed the issue of "cultural sensitivity," but their approach continues to mask structural inequalities. The focus on culture detracts attention from social, economic and political factors that exclude and trivialize the concerns of racialized minorities. Health practitioners, social service providers and policy makers have been receptive to the idea of cultural sensitivity only because it facilitates diagnoses and also masks structural factors (Ong 1995b, Watters 2001). The emphasis here is on those elements of culture (understood in static terms) that can be easily accommodated. During my field research, I observed the ease with which the Iranian New Year *(Nuroz)* was recognized and celebrated both by service providers (ESL class and recreational programmes) and the media. In an ESL class, a write-up focusing on the significance of the event was distributed to all those who were present, and the Iranian women were encouraged to display the elegant *sufre* (seven largely food dishes) for people to see and learn about this important Iranian festival. The media followed a similar line of coverage: a picture of *sufre* received emphasis, but a depoliticized write-up was mute on issues of racism and discrimination. In short, the focus was on the symbolic significance of the festival.

A conversation with a young mother reveals structural factors: "My son is so unhappy. He says his father is in Iran and we are here by ourselves on New Year. He is frustrated and unhappy." The father's stay in Iran was necessary because he could not get a job in Canada. A second example comes from an elderly woman who stated that she could no longer give money to her grandchildren, as was customary during this festival, nor did she have bus money to move around at will. Being sponsored by her son (read: dependent), she was having a difficult time financially—a state that compromised her sense of well-being. These examples reveal that cultural sensitivity cannot be translated into merely food and dance. A genuine attempt toward reaching out and being inclusive must address the issue of unequal relations of power that determine the distribution of resources and one's status in society.

Second, a focus on cultural factors places the blame on the individual for problems that have social origins. Here the script is that of "culture as a barrier." Some of the service providers informed me that elderly Iranian women do not take to physical exercises because they are inhibited by their culture. The service providers perceive these women to be "veiled" and confined to the domestic sphere. But their stories reveal that these women were active in Iran: they visited the sick, they shopped, they cooked, they maintained ties with kith and kin, and they participated in the diasporic Iranian community through travel and networking. Like the women of Deh Koh (Iran) (Friedl 1989), each woman was engaged in effecting progressive change within her own sphere of influence, however small it may have been.

In Canada, these women's ability to participate in the exercise programme was compromised by their lack of fluency in English—a situation that cannot be laid at their door. One woman stated: "I have been going to the ESL classes for four years. How come I cannot speak English?" Evidently, the woman could not learn English in the under-funded classes of four hours per week. A second issue was that the elderly women did not have money to pay the fee, even if it was as "small" as $5 for four classes. Their dependent status posed major constraints because sponsored elderly immigrants are not entitled to government benefits available to their mainstream counterparts. One elderly woman stated that she would ride the bus every day "as this was one way to fight my loneliness. When the bus fare go up, I could no longer afford to do this. I was depressed sitting at home." People on the edges of society are indeed rendered more vulnerable, as poignantly revealed in everyday life contexts. The service providers seemed to believe that the women were largely responsible for their "ill health." "They just don't want to come out. We cannot help them if they stay in their homes," said a recreational coordinator.

What we have examined above is a structural/macro-level script where the link between the mental health status of marginal social groups and societal factors is severed. But there is more to this than relegating people to a history of inattention. Within nation-states, images of marginal groups are used for political ends as seen in the well-entrenched divide between Us and Them. We are civilized and free; they are uncivilized and oppressed. This trope forms part of the colonial legacy. Referring to the Kui, a marginal community in Thailand, Das and Kleinman observe how "the colonial practice of historiography" has portrayed the community as "wild" and "as standing outside the definition of the nation and thus in need of being domesticated and brought within the agenda of national integration" (2001, 9). As is the case with other racialized minorities (Lee and Cardinal 1998), the Iranian community in Canada is rendered into a space where they are perceived as the Other. The culture and historiography of the increasingly diasporic Iranian community is barely taken into account.

Marginal groups are silenced at the most profound level possible: our society takes away the language through which these people can articulate their concerns in a manner that is meaningful to them. Despite the fact that close to 200 cultural groups are represented in Canada, this county recognizes only two Charter languages, English and French. The history of the Other cultural groups (visible minorities and First Nations people) is barely included in the school curriculum except in the way of "special topics" (Prince 2001, Beynon and Dossa 2003). As Bannerji (1995) has said, anyone who reads Canadian history would come to the conclusion that Canada has no minority groups or that if they exist they must not be significant enough to deserve mention. This form of absence has prompted scholars such as Li (2003) to make a case for the significant contributions that immigrant communities have made to Canadian society in multiple spheres of life.

The aspect of erasure of lives and non-validation of the multiple roles of Iranian women in Canada is found in all the narratives presented in this book. Sultan, Nadia, Sahra and Fatima, as well as the other research participants, take the reader on a "journey" to Iran. Their goal is to show that they lived full lives in Iran, despite the contradictions and ambiguities that surround the social and political realities of women. These women convey the message that life in Iran was not a bed of roses—for some there were more thorns than roses—but nevertheless they were in a position to struggle and negotiate the reality of their lives. These tasks were made possible because of the availability of social spaces (Friedl 1991) and female-centred kin ties (Abu-Lughod 1998). Sultan, for example, noted that the absence of these spaces in Canada has isolated her to the extent that it affects her sense of well-being and ability to settle down; Nadia discussed her domestic life to show how she dealt with the contradictions embedded in the project on modernity and gender; Sahra revealed how she held the fort in the wake of a lifetime of persecution; Fatima's example of how she was valued for her work, despite her veil, is telling.

The absence of social spaces and networks in the women's new home of Canada takes the element of struggle (hope for change) out of their lives—a hope that existed for them in Iran—and at the existential level this affects their well-being. The all-encompassing label of "refugee" made it difficult for Sultan to secure social services, tying her hands and preventing her from performing any kind of activity—even volunteer work. Structural channelling of Nadia into low-paid ghettoized work confined her to the extent that she was unable to struggle ("I have stopped struggling") as she realized that there is no hope for her to find work in her area of expertise. Sahra's lifetime struggle came to an end when she presented herself as a person who had lost the meaning of life ("When I get up in the morning, I have nothing to look forward to"). This loss came about because of her physical and social confinement, effected by her dependent status as an elderly immigrant woman. Fatima's early struggles to secure her rights as a professional working woman came to an end when she withdrew into her own niche, the export-import business. Following her daughter's car accident, Fatima entered into a new phase of life where she was left to battle on two fronts: protecting her daughter from social oppression and fighting to have her status and rights recognized as a woman, a mother and a caregiver. She refused to identify herself merely as a caregiver and she took pains to highlight the multi-faceted tasks that go along with this role. The women in this study found themselves in a position where the complicity of the larger system in their adopted country took from them the element of struggle. Yet, they did not give up but reconstructed their worlds through narratives to engage a listening community.

The women took up the challenge of making their social presence known to the outside world that had denigrated their lives and rendered them into the status of the Other. This task was made more difficult by their exclusion on multiple fronts: work, education, everyday life and other public spaces. In the eyes of the public and the media, these women are "polluting." As has been the case with other racialized minorities, the Iranians (people from the Third World) are not well received by the larger society (Bannerji 1995, Agnew 1996, Alvi 2003, Dossa 2002). Their status as Muslims is considered problematic in the wake of September 11, 2001 terrorist attack on the World Trade Center buildings in New York. As people fleeing from a revolution and the "chaos" in their own country, the Iranians are looked upon by many Canadians as "polluting" and as a "threat," given our obsession with territories and roots.

An additional factor at work is the hostility that surrounds post-revolution Iran as the establishment of the Islamic Republic exemplifies what the West fears most: Islamic fundamentalism. My conversations with Iranian women revealed that fundamentalist Islam is nuanced, a point of view also supported in critical literature (Keddie and Matthee 2002). Referring to the gendered fundamentalist ideology symbolized in the veil, one woman stated that the veil had given her more "freedom" to move around because she would not be identified. For this woman and others, the bottom line is education and work. Another woman pointed out that even in the non-fundamentalist West, women are not necessarily free.

The women in this study did not express the view that they were free in Iran. Whatever freedom they experienced was negotiated and an outcome of their kin- and peer-based networks. They regarded this form of networking as critically important. In Canada, the women are economically and socially confined, and do not feel that they have the opportunity to develop their full capacities. Their structural isolation and social invisibility deprives them of the opportunity to engage in what should be basic human rights: the right to work and to seek opportunities for social interaction. The Iranian women that I talked to emphasized that their health and sense of well-being were affected by their marginal status in Canadian society (social invisibility, structural exclusion, erasure of history and culture, and being Othered). Contrary to common wisdom, their ill health could not be attributed to their inability to adjust in a new country.

Women focused on the stories of their lives so as not to allow health practitioners and service providers to trivialize and dismiss their concerns and needs. Although many of the women had been depressed at some point during the period of re-settlement in Canada, they decided not to focus on this experience. When I engaged the women on this topic, they dismissed it: "Yes, we have experienced depression. How can we not with all the difficulties we have in this country. Our visits to the doctor have not been helpful. We don't need medication. What we need are jobs and proper English classes." Seeing that a research project had come their way, the women seized the opportunity to tell their stories and thereby give voice to their concerns. Some women, like Fatima, spoke with intensity: "I have real complains as a woman and a mother." Other women (Sahra, for example) used body language to convey their message of suffering but also that of how they are attempting to remake their worlds. The full-length stories related by four women form the core of this book. Other women who talked about particular aspects of their lives seemed to suggest that others would or could continue where they had left off; there was a common understanding that their lives converged at a point where they could speak collectively, with one voice, to challenge the dominant system that had dismissed them. One woman expressed concern that society did not consider the issues they brought forward to be important, "as if we, our lives, do not matter. It burns me inside as to how little attention is given to us as people." Each woman saw herself as participating in a collective project that redefined the common understanding of mental health and displacement.

At an early stage of my research, the female participants informed me that they did not want to talk about mental health as a series of episodes: depression, visits to the doctor, drug-therapy and its outcome. The women felt that such a focus would divide their lives into compartments and, more importantly, depoliticize the social issues responsible for their ill health. As noted earlier, the women were aware that presenting a laundry list of issues (lack of jobs, insufficient daycare, problematic English classes, racism and others) would not be an effective way to convey their message. They saw themselves as people who had been socially marginalized and hence for them the goal was to present their case in such a way that they would be heard and their lives would be socially validated. One woman stated: "I went to my social worker and told her that I wanted to attend some classes that would help me get a job. But there was no one to take care of my 5-year-old daughter. I begged her to help me find a place where I can keep my daughter for half a day. She acted as if she had not even heard me." This anecdote echoed Sultan's situation.

Raheja and Gold (1994) have argued that people who live on the margins of society know when to speak and how to present their case. While the female participants seized the research opportunity to tell their stories (consider Fatima's words: "A therapeutic chance was given to me"), they laid out the terms: the what and the how of the storytelling session. In the act of talking about their lives bifocally, they made the deliberate choice of not focusing on mental health, although I had explained to them that this was the focus of my study. Though the women did consider this to be an important issue and had all experienced compromised mental health in varying degrees, their primary interest was to establish the connection between mental health and societal factors, using two strategies.

The first one entailed a paradigm shift. The women told their stories using the social language of suffering that covers a wider expanse. By comparison, mental health evokes images of clinical encounters that individualize and medicalize essentially social issues. Also, suffering resonates more intensely with the pain that other people may have experienced in varying contexts ranging from trauma to the "soft knife of politics" (Kleinman et al. 1997, Das et al. 2000, Das et al. 2001). Through stories of suffering, the research participants problematized the equation where mental health issues are considered to arise from the trauma of displacement.

As noted earlier, our notions of displaced people are rooted in our insecurities of not belonging to and yet being territorially anchored within the body of a nation-state. These deep-rooted insecurities, as Malkki (1995) has argued, mean that displaced individuals are looked upon as "polluting" and as a "threat" to the "national order of things" (also see Gozdziak and Shandy 2000). Finding ourselves unable to categorize displaced people in what we consider to be the "natural order," we classify them as beings who need to be controlled and managed through therapy. This explains the large volume of literature on "refugee mental health."

The female participants in this study established an equation between the Iranian revolution and their uprootment. But they went further. They noted that the revolution was not brought about only by internal factors. External factors, namely foreign intervention and Western-based modernization of their country, were considered critically important. There was consensus that "were it not for the revolution, we would never have thought of leaving Iran." These women's construction of displacement was markedly different from the hegemonic construct: displacement = mental ill health. The four narratives reveal the following scenario: Sultan's account of events that led to her displacement included Germany and particularly her experience of racism in that country; the two events that led to Nadia's migration were her 16-year-old son being drafted into the military and her promise of a good job by the Canadian immigration officials; Sahra left Iran to save her husband's life; Fatima's displacement came about because she feared for her life as she was suspected of being a U.S. spy. Hence, the events that led these women to leave Iran cannot be reduced merely to the Western narrative of people from the developing world fleeing from the chaos of their own countries. To reiterate, the series of events that led to the revolution cannot be considered to be purely internal. The West has been implicated in the political developments in Iran and elsewhere in the non-Western world (Keddie 2002, Kandiyoti 1996).

A second project that the women undertook was that of re-imagining their health and well-being within the wider societal spheres of neighbourhoods, workplaces and communities—aspects that form the core elements of their narratives. The paradigm shift from an episode-based approach to mental health towards telling stories of suffering gives central space to social issues where both mental health and displacement are re-imagined in political terms.

Re-imagining Mental Health and Displacement
❧

Each of the four women in this study identified a social location from which to tell her story: that of a refugee, a woman looking for work, an aging (life-course perspective) immigrant woman or a caregiver. These social locations made it possible for these women to place issues of mental health and displacement where they belong:

in the heart of social life (political, economic, cultural and spiritual). The new understandings came about because the act of narrating a life is a means for claiming a subject position linked with the plural first person, the "we" of testimonial speaking. This aspect is revealed in the storytelling session where the participants first created a space to speak in words and through silence. The narrators also created spaces from which they could speak and potentially work towards transforming the areas of concern to them. Sultan's narrative implicates the social service sector and the refugee hearing process through a detailed account of everyday life. Her struggles in this sector, for example, her isolation, search for work, struggle for admission to programmes, and brave attempt to raise her daughter by herself—brought home her concerns and raised questions about the kind of society we live in. Through her story, Nadia raised a basic but civil rights question: "Why am I not able to find work in my area of specialization in a country that I now call home?"

The collective rendition of the above question is this: Should we not reexamine the parameters of a society that fails to meet the most basic needs of displaced persons, considering that displacement has been brought about by circumstances not of their own making? The poignancy of this question is underscored by Nadia's subversion of the hegemonic discourse on immigrant women (they cannot find work because they cannot speak English or they do not have the qualifications) and her sharing of her story as to "how she became a professional woman." We learn that this was not a linear process; Nadia's medical career was built in the context of ambiguities surrounding modernity and gender. Sahra's narrative on life-long suffering brought to light the creation of subjectivity. Sahra presented herself as a person who encountered and dealt with hardships until such time as she migrated to Canada. Here, as an aging immigrant women, her life circumstances go unnoticed. Rather than assuming a passive stance, Sahra spoke through the silent language of the body to inscribe those aspects of her life that could not be related in words, so great was her pain. Fatima buried her experience of racism in the early years of her life in Canada until she became a caregiver. She felt it necessary to relate her story: "[A] therapeutic chance ... an opportunity was given to me to review and tell out loud or let it out one of the most devastating experience a woman ... a mom may experience in her life." When she realized that society does not recognize her labour-intensive work of caregiving, she took it upon herself to become an advocate for disabled persons and caregivers. By telling her story as a mother, a woman, a caregiver and an immigrant, she positioned herself in multiple spaces where she was more likely to be heard.

The collective message that the women conveyed is that health is a human rights issue because it is the denial of their basic rights to work, to gain access to services that other citizens are entitled to, and to have their roles (for example, senior citizen or caregiver) valorized that affect their well-being and their humanity as displaced people. In their mapping of social locations of work, everyday life as a refugee, aging, and care giving, the women's stories emphasized that mental health has to do with their being and existence as women. They direct the attention of the reader and the listening community to societal barriers: downward economic mobility, racism (common sense and institutional) and general lack of opportunities to enhance their capacity to live full lives. In their narratives, the women implicated the bureaucratic practices, the ideology of the state and public spaces that compromised their sense of well-being. The women were well aware of the fact that their negative experiences in their adopted country were the result of their being Iranian/ Oriental/Other, compounded by the fact that they were displaced persons. Women that I talked to stated categorically, "Were it not for the revolution, we would not be here." Some women pointed out that the Iranian revolution was an outcome of years of Western intervention. Logically then, the West must take responsibility for these women's well-being. But such was not the case. Hence the women took it upon themselves to claim their citizenship rights in the only way possible: through re-imagining their lives using the medium of narratives that encourage the reader to question our taken-for-granted world.

Within these concrete contexts each of the woman challenged the reader to engage in a more reflexive mode that they hoped would ultimately lead to progressive change. One woman expressed it this way: "Change is brought about by rivulets. They are small and barely noticed. But imagine what would happen if they became part of the stream, and if the stream joined the river and the river joined the ocean." The women knew that their stories were the beginning of the first few and small steps—steps through which they re-imagined their worlds, not in a discrete way, but as part of a larger world. In other words, the women opposed the commonplace approach of addressing issues within ghettoized communities. This point was brought home to me during one of the storytelling sessions. After hearing the moving stories of women, a service provider said, "We should apply for funding and hire a part-time counsellor who can help these women to work through all these issues. We must make sure that the counsellor is well-qualified to do her job." The response of the Iranian women was this: "We do not need a counsellor. What we need are jobs and people that we can talk to." From their position on the margins of society, these women knew what would enhance their sense of well-being. Hence, the women ruled out the services of a part-time counsellor who would individualize their problems and deflect attention from structural barriers.

Mertz echoes the sentiments of these women even if she critiques only social science models: "[W]ork in margins and destabilized centres allows us to see through the inaccuracy of unrealistically ordered social science models and advances our understanding where more centrally located, normal-science projects have remained mired ..." (2002, 366). From within these shattered centres and vibrant margins we take the first steps towards re-imagining mental health and well-being of displaced people, keeping in mind that the displacement of the women in our study was brought about by larger forces impinging on particular stages of their life trajectories. Through the act of telling their stories of suffering, rather than discussing mental health per se, the women chalked out paths that direct us to look at the powerhouse of society that affects their lives. Because the impact is felt from the centre, change and transformation must also occur here. Insights for the direction of this change, however, must come from the position from which the cohort of our research participants speaks: the margins.

References

Abu-Lughod, Lila. 1998. "The Marriage of Feminism and Islamism in Egypt: Selective Reproduction as a Dynamic of Postcolonial Cultural Politics." In *Remaking Women Feminism and Modernity in the Middle East*, ed. Lila Abu-Lughod, 243–269. Princeton University Press.

_____, ed. 1998. *Remaking Women: Feminism and Modernity in the Middle East.* Princeton, New Jersey: Princeton University Press.

Afkhami, Mahnaz. 1994. "Women in Post-Revolutionary Iran: A Feminist Perspective." In *The Eye of the Storm: Women in Post-revolutionary Iran*, eds. Mahnaz Afkhami and Erika Friedl, 5–18. New York: Syracuse University Press.

_____, Mahnaz and Erika Friedl, eds. 1994. *In the Eye of the Storm: Women in Post-revolutionary Iran.* New York: Syracuse University Press.

Agnew, Vijay. 1996. *Resisting Discrimination: Women from Asia, Africa and the Caribbean and the Women's Movement in Canada.* Toronto: University of Toronto Press.

Ahmed, Leila. 1992. *Women and Gender in Islam: Historical Roots of a Modern Debate.* Michigan: Yale University.

Alvi, Sajida, Homa Hoodfar, and Sheila McDonough. 2003. *The Muslim Veil in North America: Issues and Debates.* Toronto: Women's Press.

Anderson, Joan. 1996. "Empowering Patients: Issues and Strategies." *Social Science and Medicine* 43 (5):697–705.

_____, Joan. 1991. "Reflexivity in Fieldwork: Towards a Feminist Epistemology." *Image: Journal of Nursing Scholarship* 23 (2):115–8.

_____, Joan, and Sheryl Kirkham. 1998. "Constructing Nation: The Gendering and Racializing of the Canadian Health Care System." In *Painting the Maple*, eds. Veronica Strong-Boag, S. Grace, A. Eisenberg, and J. Anderson, 242–261. Vancouver: UBC Press.

Appadurai, Arjun. 1991. "Global Ethnoscapes: Notes and Queries for a Transnational Anthropology." In *Recapturing Anthropology*, ed. R. Fox, 191–210. Santa Fe: School of American Research Press.

Asce, Michelle, and Adrienne Fine, eds. 1988. *Women with Disabilities: Essays in Psychology, Culture and Politics.* Philadelphia: Temple University Press.

Aylward, Carol. 1999. *Canadian Critical Race Theory: Racism and the Law*. Halifax: Fernwood Publishing.

Baha'i International Community. *The Baha'is in Iran: A Report on the Persecution of a Religious Minority*. New York: Baha'i International Community, 1981.

Bannerji, Himani. 2001. *Inventing Subjects: Studies in Hegemony, Patriarchy and Colonialism*. New Delhi: Tulika Print Communication Services Pvt. Ltd.

_____, Himani. 2000. *The Dark Side of the Nation: Essays on Multiculturalism, Nationalism and Gender*. Toronto, Canada: Canadian Scholars' Press.

_____, Himani. 1995. *Thinking Through: Essays on Feminism, Marxism, and Anti-Racism*. Toronto: Women's Press.

Becker, Gay. 1997. *Disrupted Lives: How People Create Meaning in a Chaotic World*. Berkeley: University of California Press.

Behar, Ruth. 1996. *The Vulnerable Observer: Anthropology that Breaks Our Heart*. Boston: Beacon Press.

_____, Ruth, and Deborah A. Gordon, eds. 1995. *Women Writing Culture*. Berkeley: University of California Press.

Beverley, Joan 1992. "The Margin at the Center: On Testimonio (Testimonial Narrative)." In *De/Colonizing the Subject*, eds. S. Smith and J. Watson, 91–114. Minneapolis: University of Minnesota Press.

Beynon, June, and Parin Dossa. 2003. "Mapping Inclusive and Equitable Pedagogy: Narratives of University Educators." *Teacher Education* 14 (3):253–264.

Bonny, Norton. 2000. *Identity and Language Learning: Gender, Ethnicity and Educational Practice*. New York: Longman.

Boyd, Monica 1992. "Gender, Visible Minority and Immigrant Earnings Inequality: Reassessing and Employment Equity Premise." Department Working Paper. Department of Sociology and Anthropology. Ottawa: Carleton University.

British Columbia Newcomers' Guide to Resources and Services. 2000. Vancouver: Ministry of Multiculturalism and Immigration.

Canadian Task Force on Mental Health. 1988. *Issues Affecting Immigrants and Refugees: Review of the Literature on Migrant Mental Health*. Ottawa: Ministry of Supply and Services.

Casey, Kathleen. 1993. *I Answer with My Life: Life Histories of Women Teachers Working for Social Change*. New York: Routledge.

Chuengsatiansup, Komatra. 2001. "Marginality, Suffering and Community: The Politics of Collective Experience and Empowerment in Thailand." In *Remaking a World: Violence, Social Suffering and Recovery*, eds. Veena Das et al., 31–73. Berkeley: University of California Press.

Collins, Patricia Hill. 2000. *Black Feminist Thought: Knowledge, Consciousness, and the Politics of Empowerment*, 2nd edition. 1990. New York: Routledge.

Corker, Mairian and Sally French. 1999. "Reclaiming Discourse in Disability Studies." In *Disability Discourse*, eds. Mairian Corker and Sally French, 1–12. Philadelphia: Open University Press.

Creese, Gillian. 1992. "The Politics of Refugees in Canada." In *Deconstructing a Nation: Immigration, Multiculturalism and Racism in 90s Canada*, ed. Vic Satzewich, 123–144. Halifax, Nova Scotia: Fernwood Publishing.

Cruikshank, Julie. 1998. *The Social Life of Stories: Narrative and Knowledge in the Yukon Territory*. Vancouver: University of British Columbia Press.

REFERENCES

Das, Veena, and Arthur Kleinman. 2001. "Introduction." In *Remaking a World: Violence, Social Suffering, and Recovery*, eds. V. Das et al., 1–30. Berkeley: University of California Press.

_____, Veena, Arthur Kleinman, M. Ramphele, and P. Reynolds, eds. 2000. *Violence and Subjectivity*. Berkeley: University of California Press.

De Groot, Joanna. 1996. "Gender, Discourse and Ideology in Iranian Studies: Towards a New Scholarship." In *Gendering the Middle East: Emerging Perspectives*, ed. Deniz Kandiyoti, 20–50. Syracuse, New York: Syracuse University Press.

Devault, M. 1990. "Talking and Listening from Women's Standpoint: Feminist Strategies for Interviewing and Analysis." *Social Problems* 37 (1):96–116.

Dossa, Parin. 2002a. "Narrative Mediation of Conventional and New Mental Health Paradigms: Reading the Stories of Immigrant Iranian Women." *Medical Anthropology Quarterly* 16 (3):341–359.

_____, Parin. 2002b. "Reconfiguring the Question: Who Is a Refugee? Coming to Voice, Coming to Power: One Woman's Story." *Pakistani Journal on Women's Studies* 9 (1):27–55.

_____, Parin. 2000. "On Law and Hegemonic Moments: Looking Beyond the Law Towards Subjectivities of Subaltern Women." In *Law as Gendering Practice: Canadian Perspectives*, eds. Dorothy E. Chunn and Dany Lacome, 138–57. Don Mills, Ontario: Oxford University Press.

_____, Parin. 1999. "(Re)imagining Aging Lives: Ethnographic Narratives of Muslim Women in Diaspora." *Journal of Cross-Cultural Gerontology* 14 (3):245–272.

Douglas, Mary. 1966. *Purity and Danger: An Analysis of the Concepts of Pollution and Taboo.* London: Routledge.

Dua, Enakshi, and Angela Robertson. 1999. "Introduction." In *Scratching the Surface: Canadian Anti-Racist Feminist Thought*, 7–33. Toronto: Women's Press.

Dyck, Isabel. 1998. "Methodologies on the Line: Constructing Meanings about 'Cultural Difference' in Health Care Research." In *Painting the Maple: Essays on Race, Gender and the Construction of Canada*, eds. V. Strong-Boad et al., 19–36. Vancouver: UBC Press.

_____, Isabel. 1995. "Putting Chronic Illness 'in Place': Women Immigrants' Accounts of their Health Care." *Geoforum* 26:247–60.

Escobar, Arturo. 1995. *Encountering Development: The Making and Unmaking of the Third World.* Princeton: Princeton University Press.

Estes, Carol. 1979. *The Aging Enterprise: A Critical Examination of Social Policies and Services for the Aged.* San Francisco: Jossey-Bass Publishers.

Fahmy, Khaled. 1998. "Women, Medicine, and Power in Nineteenth-Century Egypt." In *Remaking Women: Feminism and Modernity in the Middle East*, ed. Lila Abu-Lughod, 35–72. Princeton, New Jersey: Princeton University Press.

Farmer, Paul. 2003. *Pathologies of Power: Health, Human Rights, and the New War on the Poor.* Berkeley: University of California Press.

Farr, Grant. 1999. *Modern Iran.* Boston: McGraw-Hill College.

Fernando, Tisa. 1979. "East African Asians in Western Canada: The Ismaili Community." *New Community* 7 (3):361–368.

Foster, Lorne. 1998. *Turnstile Immigration: Multiculturalism, Social Order and Social Justice in Canada.* Toronto: Thompson Education Publishing.

Foucault, Michel. 1978. *History of Sexuality.* Pantheon: New York.

_____, Michel. 1973. *The Birth of the Clinic: An Archeology of Medical Perception.* Pantheon: New York.

Fox-Genovese, Elizabeth. 1991. *Feminism Without Illusions: A Critique of Individualism.* Chapel Hill: University of North Carolina Press.

Frank, Arthur. 1995. *The Wounded Story Teller.* Chicago: The University of Chicago Press.

Frank, Gelya. 2000. *Venus on Wheels: Two Decades of Dialogue on Disability, Biography, and Being Female in America.* Berkeley: University of California Press.

Fraser, Nancy. 1989. *Unruly Practices: Power, Discourse and Gender in Contemporary Social Theory.* Minneapolis: University of Minnesota Press.

French, Lindsay. 1994. "The Political Economy of Injury and Compassion: Amputees on the Thai Cambodian Border." In *Embodiment and Experience: The Existential Ground of Culture and Self,* ed. Thomas I. Csordas, 69–99. Cambridge: Cambridge University Press.

Friedl, Erika. 1991. "The Dynamics of Women's Spheres of Action in Rural Iran." In *Women in Middle Eastern History: Shifting Boundaries in Sex and Gender,* eds. N. Keddie and B. Baron, 195–214. Binghamton: Vail-Ballou Press.

_____, Erika. 1989. *Women of Deh Koh: Lives in an Iranian Village.* Washington: Smithsonian Institution Press.

Gal, Susan 1991. "Between Speech and Silence: The Problematics of Research on Language and Gender." In *Gender at the Crossroads of Knowledge: Feminist Anthropology in the Postmodern Era,* ed. M. Leonardo, 175–203. Berkeley: University of California Press.

Good, Byron. 1994. *Medicine, Rationality, and Experience.* New York: Cambridge University Press.

_____, Byron. 1977. "The Heart of What's the Matter: The Semantics of Illness in Iran." *Culture, Medicine and Psychiatry* 1:25–8.

Good, M. Delvecchio, P. E. Broadwin, B. Good, and A. Kleinman. eds. 1992. *Pain as Human Experience: An Anthropological Perspective.* Berkeley: University of California Press.

Gozdziak, Elzbieta, and Dianna Shandy, eds. 2000. *Rethinking Refugee and Displacement.* Selected Papers on Refugees and Immigrants, vol. viii. Arlington, VA: American Anthropological Association.

Greenhouse, Carol, Elizabeth Mertz, and Kay Warren, eds. 2002. *Ethnography in Unstable Places: Everyday Lives in Contexts of Dramatic Political Change.* Durham and London: Duke University Press.

Guha, Ranjit. 1996. *The Small Voice of History In Subaltern Studies IX: Writings on South Asian History and Society,* eds. S. Amin and D. Chakrabarty, 1–12. Delhi: Oxford University Press.

Gupta, Tania D. 1996. *Racism and Paid Work.* Toronto: Garamond Press.

Harrison, Fay. 1997. "The Gendered Politics and Violence of Structural Adjustment." In *Situated Lives: Gender and Culture in Everyday Life,* eds. L. Lamphere, H. Ragone, and P. Zavella, 451–68. New York: Routledge.

Henry, Frances, C. Tator, W. Mattis, and T. Rees. 1995. *The Colour of Democracy: Racism in Canadian Society.* Toronto: Harcourt Brace Canada.

Hoodfar, Homa. 1997. *Between Marriage and the Market: Intimate Politics and Survival in Cairo.* Berkeley: University of California Press.

REFERENCES

Hyndman, Jennifer. 1999. "Gender and Canadian Immigration Policy: A Current Snapshot." *Canadian Woman Studies* 19 (3):6–10.

Ingstad, Benedicte, and Susan Whyte. 1995. *Disability and Culture.* Berkeley: University of California Press.

Jiwani, Yasmin. 2001. *Intersecting Inequalities: Immigrant Women of Colour, Violence and Health Care.* Vancouver: Feminist Research, Education, Development and Action.

Joseph, Suad, and Susan Slyomovics, eds. 2001. *Women and Power in the Middle East.* Philadelphia: University of Pennsylvania Press.

Kandiyoti, Deniz, ed. 1996. *Gendering the Middle East: Emerging Perspectives.* Syracuse: Syracuse University Press.

Kazemzadeh, Firuz. 2002. The Baha'is in Iran: Twenty Years of Repression. *Social Research* 67 (2):537–557.

Keddie, Nikki, and Beth Baron. 1991. "Introduction: Deciphering Middle Eastern History." In *Women in Middle Eastern History: Shifting Boundaries in Sex and Gender,* eds. N. Keddie and Beth Baron, 1–29. Binghamton, New York: Vail-Ballour Press.

_____, Nikki, and Rudi Matthee eds. 2002. *Iran and the Surrounding World: Interactions in Culture and Cultural Politics.* Seattle: University of Washington.

Kleinman, Arthur. 1988. *The Illness Narratives: Suffering, Health and the Human Condition.* New York: Basic Books.

_____, Arthur, and Joan Kleinman, eds. 1997. "The Appeal of Experience; The Dismay of Images: Cultural Appropriation of Suffering in Our Times." In *Social Suffering,* eds. A. Kleinman et al., 1–24. Berkeley: University of California Press.

_____, Arthur, Margaret Lock, and Veena Das, eds. 1997. "Introduction." In *Social Suffering,* ix–xxvii. Berkeley: University of California Press.

Krulfeld, Ruth, and Linda Camino. 1994. "Introduction." In *Reconstructing Lives, Recapturing Meaning: Refugee Identity, Gender, and Culture Change,* eds. Linda Camino and Ruth Krulfeld, ix–xviii. Postfach, Switzerland: Gordon and Breach Publishers.

Kumar, Amitava. 2000. *Passport Photos.* Berkeley: University of California Press.

Lamb, Sarah. 2000. *White Saris and Sweet Mangoes: Aging, Gender, and Body in North India.* Berkeley: University of California Press.

Lee, Jo-Anne. 1999. "Immigrant Women Workers in the Immigrant Settlement Sector." *Canadian Woman Studies* 19 (3):97–103.

_____, Jo-Anne, and Linda Cardinal. 1998. "Hegemonic Nationalism and the Politics of Feminism and Multiculturalism in Canada." In *Painting the Maple: Essays on Race, Gender, and the Construction of Canada,* eds. Veronica Strong-Boag, S. Grace, A. Eisenberg, and J. Anderson, 215–241. Vancouver: UBC Press.

Li, Peter. 2003. *Destination Canada: Immigration Debates and Issues.* Don Mills, Ontario: Oxford University Press.

Lindenbaum, Shirley, and Margaret Lock. 1993. *Knowledge, Power, and Practice: The Anthropology of Medicine and Everyday Life.* Berkeley: University of California Press.

Lippard, Lucy, ed. 1992. *Partial Recall: With Essays on Photographs of Native Americans.* New York: The New Press.

Lipson, J. 1992. "The Health and Adjustment of Iranian Immigrants." *Western Journal of Nursing Research* 14(1):10–29.

Lock, Margaret. 1993. *Encounters with Aging: Mythologies of Menopause in Japan and North America*. Berkeley: University of California Press.

_____, Margaret, and Patricia Kaufert. 1998. "Introduction." In *Pragmatic Women and Body Politics*, 1–27. New York: Cambridge University Press.

Malkki, Liisa. 1995. *Purity and Exile: Violence, Memory and National Cosmology Among Hutu Refugees in Tanzania*. Chicago: The University of Chicago Press.

McGowan, Rima. 1999. *Muslims in the Diaspora: The Somali Communities of London and Toronto*. Toronto: University of Toronto Press.

Melotti, Umberto. 1997. "International Migration in Europe: Social Projects and Political Cultures." In *The Politics of Multiculturalism in the New Europe: Racism, Identity and Community*, ed. Tariq Modood and Panina Werbner, 73–92. New York: Zed Books.

Mernissi, Fatima. 1991. *Women and Islam: An Historical and Theological Inquiry*, trans. M. Lakeland. Oxford: Blackwell.

_____, Fatima. 1975. *Beyond the Veil: Male-Female Dynamics in a Modern Muslim Society*. New York: Halsted Press.

Mertz, Elizabeth. 2002. "The Perfidy of Gaze and the Pain of Uncertainty: Anthropological Theory and the Search for Closure." In *Ethnography in Unstable Places*, eds. Greenhouse et al., 355–78. Durham and London: Duke University Press.

Milani, Farzaneh. 1992. *Veils and Words: The Emerging Voices of Iranian Women Writers*. New York: Syracuse University Press.

Minh-ha, Trinh T. 1989. *Woman Native Other*. Bloomington: Indiana University Press.

Mitrovica, Andrew. 2000. "Refugee Claimants Inundate Ontario." *Globe and Mail* (11 December).

Modood, Tariq. 1997. "Introduction: The Politics of Multiculturalism in the New Europe." In *The Politics of Multiculturalism in the New Europe: Racism, Identity and Community*, eds. Tariq Modood and Panina Werbner, 1–26. New York: Zed Books.

Moghadam, Fatemeh. 1994. "Commoditization of Sexuality and Female Labor Participation in Islam: Implications for Iran, 1960–90." In *The Eye of the Storm*, eds. Mahnaz Afkhami and Erika Friedl, 80–97. London: I. B. Tauris.

Mohanty, Chandra. 2003. *Feminism Without Borders: Decolonizing Theory, Practicing Solidarity*. Durham: Duke University Press.

Monks, Judith, and Ronald Frankenberg. 1995. "Being Ill and Being Me: Self, Body, and Time in Multiple Sclerosis Narratives." In *Disability and Culture*, eds. B. Ingstad and S. Whyte, 107–134. Berkeley: University of California Press.

Moore, Henrietta. 1996. *The Future of Anthropological Knowledge*. New York: Routledge.

_____, Henrietta. 1988. *Feminism and Anthropology*. Minneapolis: University of Minnesota Press.

_____, Henrietta, ed. 2000. *Anthropological Theory Today*. Cambridge: Polity Press.

Morrow, Marina, and Monika Chappell. 1999. *Hearing Women's Voices: Mental Health Care for Women*. Vancouver, B.C: British Columbia Centre of Excellence for Women's Health.

Myerhoff, Barbara, and Andrea Simic, eds. 1978. *Life's Career Aging: Cultural Variations on Growing Old*. Newbury Park, California: Sage Publications.

Naples, Nancy, and Manisha Desai, eds. 2002. *Women's Activism and Globalization: Linking Local Struggles and Transnational Politics*. New York: Routledge.

Nashat, Guity, and Judith Tucker. 1999. *Women in the Middle East and North Africa: Restoring Women to History*. Bloomington: Indiana University Press.

Najmabadi, Afsaneh. 1998a. "Crafting an Educated Housewife in Iran." In *Remaking Women: Feminism and Modernity in the Middle East*, ed. Lila Abu-Lughod, 91–125. Princeton, New Jersey: Princeton University Press.

_____, Afsaneh. 1998b. *The Story of the Daughters of Quchan: Gender and National Memory in Iranian History*. New York: Syracuse University Press.

Ng, Roxana. 1996. *The Politics of Community Services: Immigrant Women, Class and State*, 2nd edition. 1988. Toronto, Ontario: Garamond Press.

Norton, Bonny. 2000. *Identity and Language Learning: Social Processes and Education Practice*. Essex, U.K.: Pearson Education.

Oliver, Michael. 1996. *Understanding Disability: From Theory to Practice*. Basingstoke: Macmillan.

Ong, Aihwa. 1999. *Flexible Citizenship: The Cultural Logics of Transnationality*. London: Duke University Press.

_____, Aihwa. 1995a. "Women out of China: Travelling Tales and Travelling Theories in Postcolonial Feminism." In *Women Writing Culture*, eds. Ruth Behar and Deborah Gordon, 350–372. Berkeley: University of California Press.

_____, Aihwa. 1995b. "Making the Biopolitical Subject: Cambodian Immigrants, Refugee Medicine and Cultural Citizenship in California." *Social Science and Medicine* 40 (9):1243–57.

_____, Aihwa. 1987. *Spirits of Resistance and Capitalist Discipline: Factory Women in Malaysia*. Albany: State University of New York Press.

Opie, Anne. 1992. *There's Nobody There: Community Care of Confused Older People*. New Zealand: Oxford University Press.

Ortner, Sherry. 1994. "Theory in Anthropology Since the Sixties." In *Culture/Power/History: A Reading in Contemporary Social Theory*, eds. N. B. Dirks, G. Eley, and S. B. Ortner, 372–411. Princeton: Princeton University Press.

Personal Narratives Group, eds. 1989. *Interpreting Women's Lives: Feminist Theory and Personal Narratives*. Bloomington: Indiana University Press.

Pliskin, K. 1987. *Silent Boundaries: Cultural Constraints on Sickness and Diagnoses of Iranians in Israel*. New Haven: Yale University Press.

Prince, Althea. 2001. *Being Black: Essays*. Toronto: Insomniac Press.

Puar, Jasbir. 1994. "Writing My Way 'Home': Traveling South Asian bodies and Diasporic Journeys." *Socialist Review* 24 (4):75–108.

Raheja, Gloria, and Ann Gold. 1994. *Listen to the Heron's Words: Reimagining Gender and Kinship in North India*. Berkeley: University of California Press.

Ram, Kalpana, and Margaret Jolly. 1998. *Maternities and Modernities: Colonial and Postcolonial Experiences in Asia and the Pacific*. Cambridge: Cambridge University Press.

Razack, Sherene. 1998. *Looking White People in the Eye: Gender, Race, and Culture in Courtrooms and Classrooms*. Toronto: University of Toronto Press.

Rodriguez, Carmen. 1997. *And a Body to Remember With*. Vancouver, BC: Arsenal Pulp Press.

Ross, Fiona. 2001. "Speech and Silence: Women's Testimony in the First Five Weeks of Public Hearings of the South African Truth and Reconciliation Commission." In

Remaking a World, eds. Veena Das et al., 250–80. Berkeley: University of California Press.

Said, Edward. 1978. *Orientalism*. New York: Vintage Books.

Scheper-Hughes, Nancy. 1992. *Death Without Weeping: The Violence of Everyday Life in Brazil*. Berkeley: University of California Press.

Smith, Dorothy. 1999. *Writing the Social: Critique, Theory and Investigation*. Toronto: University of Toronto Press.

———, Dorothy. 1987. *The Everyday World As Problematic: A Feminist Sociology*. Boston: Northeastern University Press.

———, Dorothy. 1984. *The Renaissance of Women: Knowledge Reconsidered: A Feminist Overview*. Canadian Research Institute for the Advancement of Women. Ottawa: CRIAW Publications Committee.

Spivak, Gayatri Chakravorty. 1988. *Can the Subaltern Speak? Marxism and the Interpretation of Culture*, eds. C. Nelson and L. Gossberg, 217–313. Urbana: University of Illinois Press.

Stevenson, Winona 1999. "Colonialism and First Nations Women in Canada." In *Scratching the Surface*, eds. Enakshi Dua and Angela Robertson, 49–80. Toronto: Women's Press.

Sullivan, Zohreh 1998. "Eluding the Feminist, Overthrowing the Modern? Transformations in Twentieth-Century Iran." In *Remaking Women: Feminism and Modernity in the Middle East*, ed. Lila Abu-Lughod, 215–42. Princeton, New Jersey: Princeton University Press.

Taherzadeh, A. *The Covenant of Baha'ullah*. Oxford: G. Ronald, 1992.

Taylor, Charles. 1994. *Multiculturalism: Examining the Politics of Recognition*. Princeton, New Jersey: Princeton University Press.

Thobani, Sunera. 1999. "Sponsoring Immigrant Women's Inequalities." *Canadian Woman Studies* 19 (3):11–17.

Tinker, Irene. 1997. *Street Foods: Urban Food and Employment in Developing Countries*. Oxford: Oxford University Press.

Todeschini, Maya. 2001. "The Bomb's Womb? Women and the Atom Bomb." In *Remaking a World*, eds. Veena Das et al., 102–156. Berkeley: University of California Press.

Turner, Victor. 1967. *The Forest of Symbols: Aspects of Ndembu Ritual*. Ithaca, New York: Cornell University Press.

Van Gennep. 1960. *The Rites of Passage*. Chicago: University of Chicago Press.

Visweswaran, Kamala. 1994. *Fictions of Feminist Anthropology*. Minneapolis: The University of Minnesota Press.

Watters, Charles. 2001. "Emerging Paradigms in the Mental Health Care of Refugees." *Social Science and Medicine* 52:1709–18.

Wendell, Susan. 1996. *The Rejected Body: Feminist Philosophical Reflections on Disability*. New York: Routledge.

Whyte, Susan, and Benedicte Ingstad. 1995. "Disability and Culture: An Overview." In *Disability and Culture*, eds. Ingstad Benedicte and Susan Whyte, 3–37. Berkeley: University of California Press.

Wolf, Diane L. 1996. "Situating Feminist Dilemmas in Fieldwork." In *Feminist Dilemmas in Fieldwork*, ed. Diane L. Wolf, 1–55. Boulder: Westview Press.

Yuval-Davis, N. 1997. *Gender and Nation*. London: Sage Publications.

Index